THE UNIVERSITY OF MAINE
AT AUGUSTA

STUDENT AGGRESSION

Student Aggression
Prevention, Management, and Replacement Training

ARNOLD P. GOLDSTEIN
BERJ HAROOTUNIAN
JANE CLOSE CONOLEY

THE GUILFORD PRESS
New York   London

©1994 The Guilford Press
A Division of Guilford Publications, Inc.
72 Spring Street, New York, NY 10012

Printed in the United States of America

This book is printed on acid-free paper.

Last digit is print number: 9 8 7 6 5 4 3 2

Library of Congress Cataloging-in-Publication Data

Goldstein, Arnold P.
    Student aggression : prevention, management, and replacement
training / Arnold P. Goldstein, Berj Harootunian, and Jane Close
Conoley.
      p. cm.
    Includes bibliographicial references and index.
    ISBN 0-89862-246-8
    1. School violence—United States. 2. School discipline—United
States. 3. Problem children—Education—United States.
I. Harootunian, Berj. II. Conoley, Jane Close. III. Title.
LB3013.3.G65   1994
371.5'8—dc20
                                                                 93-34735
                                                                     CIP

In the early 1980s, we three and a fourth colleague, Steven J. Apter, began a series of collaborations concerned with children, schools, and means for their effective partnership. What were then termed "disturbed and disturbing" youngsters was the focus of *Childhood Behavior Disorders and Emotional Disturbance* (Apter & Conoley, 1984). School violence and vandalism, circa 1984, was the concern of *School Violence* (Goldstein, Apter, & Harootunian, 1984). The present book incorporates the ecological and empirical spirit of both these earlier monographs, and some of the content of the latter, serving as a springboard, as it were, to explore and examine in depth the efforts of the last decade to prevent, manage, and replace student aggression in the contemporary school.

+

Steve Apter died in 1985. With the fondest remembrance of a most special colleague, collaborator, and friend, we dedicate this book to him.

Contents

INTRODUCTION

The Problem

Aggression and America are long-term and intimate companions. Collective and individual aggression have been and continue to be prominent features of the American scene. Collective aggression, born in a frontier spirit and enhanced by both the sanctioned collective aggression of warfare and the ready availability of guns in the United States, has historically found diverse expression in vigilante movements, feuding, agrarian and labor strife, racial lynchings, student and antiwar riots and, in recent years, in ever-increasing levels of youth gang violence. Individual aggression in America is more difficult to place in historical perspective for two reasons. First, the major means of systematically recording and enumerating individual criminal acts in the United States, the Federal Bureau of Investigation's *Uniform Crime Reports,* were not used until 1933. Thus, less systematic and comprehensive historical accounts must be relied on for information regarding pre-1933 levels of criminal aggression in America. Second, certain other forms of individual aggression, notably child and spouse abuse and a few classes of juvenile "misbehavior," were not a matter of general public concern and attention until the late 1960s. Such societal indifference to these behaviors has changed dramatically in recent years.

   Much of what can be reported factually about recent trends in individual aggression, especially of a criminal nature, is depicted in Table 1.1. This table, drawn from the FBI's *Uniform Crime Reports* for 1981 through 1990, is derived from crime statistics voluntarily submitted to the FBI by police departments across America. It shows both the number and the rate per 100,000 inhabitants of major violent and property crimes in the United States. Violent crimes include murder, forcible

TABLE 1.1. Index of Crime, United States, 1981–1990

	Crime index total	Violent crime	Property crime	Murder and nonnegligent manslaughter	Forcible rape	Robbery	Aggravated assault	Burglary	Larceny-theft	Motor vehicle theft
				Number of offenses						
Population by year:										
1981: 229,146,000	13,423,800	1,361,820	12,061,900	22,520	82,500	592,910	663,900	3,779,700	7,194,400	1,087,800
1982: 231,534,000	12,974,400	1,322,390	11,652,000	21,010	78,770	553,130	669,480	3,447,100	7,142,500	1,062,400
1983: 233,981,000	12,108,600	1,258,090	10,850,500	19,310	78,920	506,570	653,290	3,129,900	6,712,800	1,007,900
1984: 236,158,000	11,881,800	1,273,280	10,608,500	18,690	84,230	485,010	685,350	2,984,400	6,591,900	1,032,200
1985: 238,740,000	12,431,400	1,328,800	11,102,600	18,980	88,670	497,870	723,250	3,073,300	6,926,400	1,102,900
1986: 241,077,000	13,211,900	1,489,170	11,722,700	20,610	91,460	542,780	834,320	3,241,400	7,257,200	1,224,100
1987: 243,400,000	13,508,700	1,484,000	12,024,700	20,100	91,110	517,700	855,090	3,236,200	7,499,900	1,288,700
1988: 245,807,000	13,923,100	1,566,220	12,356,900	20,680	92,490	542,970	910,090	3,218,100	7,705,900	1,432,900
1989: 248,239,000	14,251,400	1,646,040	12,605,400	21,500	94,500	578,330	951,710	3,168,200	7,872,400	1,564,800
1990: 248,709,873	14,475,600	1,820,130	12,655,500	23,440	102,560	639,270	1,054,860	3,073,900	7,945,700	1,635,900
Percent change in number of offenses:										
1990/1989	+1.6	+10.6	+0.4	+9.0	+8.5	+10.5	+10.8	−3.0	+0.9	+4.5
1990/1986	+9.6	+22.2	+8.0	+13.7	+12.1	+17.8	+26.4	−5.2	+9.5	+33.6
1990/1981	+7.8	+33.7	+4.9	+4.1	+24.3	+7.8	+58.9	−18.7	+10.4	+50.4
				Rate per 100,000 inhabitants						
Year:										
1981	5,858.2	594.3	5,263.9	9.8	36.0	258.7	289.7	1,649.5	3,139.7	474.7
1982	5,603.6	571.1	5,032.5	9.1	34.0	238.9	289.2	1,488.8	3,084.8	458.8
1983	5,175.0	537.7	4,637.4	8.3	33.7	216.5	279.2	1,337.7	2,868.9	430.8
1984	5,031.3	539.2	4,492.1	7.9	35.7	205.4	290.2	1,263.7	2,791.3	437.1
1985	5,207.1	556.6	4,650.5	7.9	37.1	208.5	302.9	1,287.3	2,901.2	462.0
1986	5,480.4	617.7	4,862.6	8.6	37.9	225.1	346.1	1,344.6	3,010.3	507.8
1987	5,550.0	609.7	4,940.3	8.3	37.4	212.7	351.3	1,329.6	3,081.3	529.9
1988	5,664.2	637.2	5,027.1	8.4	37.6	220.9	370.2	1,309.2	3,134.9	582.9
1989	5,741.0	663.1	5,077.9	8.7	38.1	233.0	383.4	1,276.3	3,171.3	630.4
1990	5,820.3	731.8	5,088.5	9.4	41.2	257.0	424.1	1,235.9	3,194.8	657.8
Percent change in rate per 100,000 inhabitants:										
1990/1989	+1.4	+10.4	+0.2	+8.0	+8.1	+10.3	+10.6	−3.2	+0.7	+4.3
1990/1986	+6.2	+18.5	+4.6	+9.3	+8.7	+14.2	+22.5	−8.1	+6.1	+29.5
1990/1981	−0.6	+23.1	−3.3	−4.1	+14.4	−0.7	+46.4	−25.1	+1.8	+38.6

Note. Adapted from Federal Bureau of Investigation (1989, 1990).

rape, robbery, and aggravated assault; property crimes include burglary, larceny/theft, and motor vehicle theft. These data provide a context for the more specific examination of similarly aggressive behaviors in a school setting that is to follow. We think the understanding of school violence requires such placement in societal context, since the levels, forms, and causes of aggression by youths in America's schools appear to parallel and reflect the levels, forms, and causes of aggression in our society at large.

The statistical levels and trends depicted in Table 1.1 are the focus of considerable attention and often diverse interpretation in the United States. We understand these data, as does Skogan (1989), to mean that crime in America increased in a consistent manner during the period, with the exception of a minor, transitory dip at mid-decade. Skogan (1989) summarizes the picture accurately:

> Those [diverse national] data portray steadily increasing rates of violence in the United States since the mid-1950s. The rate of violent crime [murder, rape, robbery, aggravated assault] rose slowly between then and near the middle of the 1960s, but it rose without interruption every year. Between 1955 and 1975, levels of violent crime increased by a factor of more than four; the property crime rate followed almost exactly the same pattern. Then, there was a three-year respite in this trend, a brief period during which both violent and property crime rates leveled off at nearly their 1975 high; this was followed by a climb to a new high in 1982, and again in 1986. Between 1953 and 1986, the violent crime rate rose almost exactly 600 percent and the property crime rate 400 percent. (p. 236)

Such heightened violence has become especially acute for America's young people. Between 1981 and 1990, all categories of violent crime increased substantially for youths under age 18: murder and non-negligent manslaughter (60.1%), forcible rape (28.2%), and aggravated assault (56.5%), an overall violent crime increase of 29.1% (FBI, 1990). Of those persons in the United States arrested for violent crimes in 1990, 23,060 were under age 15, and 1,270 were younger than 10.

Anecdotal evidence strongly suggests that this increase in youth violence is occurring for both males and females ("Youth Violence," 1991). One of every 10 American youngsters who died in 1987 was killed with a gun. In both 1988 (with 1,538 deaths) and 1989 (with 1,897 deaths), new records for firearm murders of youths 19 and under were established in the United States. These dramatic increases hold when adjusted for population growth ("Caught in the Crossfire," 1990). Teenagers in America were, at minimum, at least four times as likely to be murdered than were their counterparts in 21 other industrialized counries. It is worth noting that there are approximately 200 million privately owned guns in the United States. In 1990 alone, 1.8 million pistols and revolvers were manufactured in the United States, and 683,000 handguns were imported ("Youth Violence," 1992).

The American home is no stranger to physical aggression. A nationwide survey conducted in 1968 for the National Commission on the Causes and Prevention of Violence (Mulvihill, Tumin, & Curtis, 1969) revealed that 93% of survey respondents reported having been spanked in childhood; 55% had been slapped or kicked, 31% punched or beaten, 14% threatened or cut with a knife, and 12% threatened with a gun or shot at. Domestic violence is visited not only upon children; spouses, particularly wives, are also frequent targets of physical abuse. Strauss (1977, 1978) estimates that approximately 25% of wives have been targets of physical aggression by their husbands, an estimate generally reaffirmed in subsequent analyses (e.g., Stark & Flitcraft, 1988). An equally grim picture emerges for elderly citizens. In 1990, the United States House of Representatives Subcommittee on Health and Long-Term Care reported that 1.5 million elderly Americans, or 5% of all elderly U.S. citizens, are physically abused each year, most by their own children. In 1980, the comparable estimate was 1 million ("Elderly Abuse," 1990).

The recent history of child abuse in the United States has followed a parallel path. As recently as the mid-1960s, the terms "child abuse" and "battered child syndrome" were not part of either public or professional awareness. Largely through the efforts of such persons as Gil (1970), Helfer and Kempe (1976), and Kempe, Silverman, Steele, Droegemueller, and Silver (1962), significant consciousness raising has occurred. The nation is now keenly aware of child abuse. The number of child abuse incidents is substantial, reported in 1984 to be 1.7 million, an increase of 17% from 1983 and 158% from 1976, the first year such data were systematically collected (American Humane Society, 1986). Subsequent years continue to show a steady rise in the number of children reportedly abused: 1.9 million in 1985, 2.0 million in 1986, 2.1 million in 1987, 2.2 million in 1988, and 2.4 million in 1989 (Federation of Child Abuse and Neglect, 1990).

In addition to streets and homes, the United States' third major setting for the expression of aggressive behavior is its mass media: newspapers, books, comics, radio, movies, and especially television. The impact of the contemporary mass media on behavior is immense, one manifestation of which has been an increase in violence. This assertion is still in dispute, but a reading of the evidence showing the influence of television viewing on overt aggression in particular leaves little room for doubt or equivocation (Comstock, 1983). The heavy diet of violence offered by television appears to contribute substantially to both the acquisition of aggressive behavior and the instigation of its enactment.

Prime time television in the United States during 1989 showed an average of 9.5 acts of violence per hour. The comparable figure for 1982 was 7 such acts per hour. Saturday morning cartoons now portray 25 violent acts per hour. By age 16, the average adolescent—who views approximately 35 hours of television programming per week—will have seen 200,000 acts of violence, 33,000 of which are murders or attempted murders (National Coalition on Television Violence, 1990). No wonder a substantial minority of viewers will engage in copycat violence.

The pernicious effects of television violence go further, as they extend to the substantial decrease in sensitivity, concern, and revulsion toward violence among the viewing audience. Higher and higher levels of violence become more and more tolerable. These and other aggression-enhancing and aggression-tolerating effects of television have been documented in many sources (Baker & Ball, 1969; Brown, 1976; Comstock, 1983, 1992; Feshbach & Singer, 1971; Howitt & Cumberbatch, 1975; Lefkowitz, Eron, Walder, & Huessman, 1977; Liebert, Neale, & Davidson, 1973).

While the levels and forms of aggression so evident in our streets, homes, and mass media provide context for our view of aggression in America's schools, acts of school violence are best viewed not as a phenomenon apart, but as yet another manifestation of behavioral trends that characterize so much of contemporary life in the United States.

AGGRESSION TOWARD PERSONS

In American public education during the decades preceding the 20th century, aggression in schools toward either people or property was infrequent in occurrence, low in intensity, and—at least in retrospect— almost quaint in character. "Misbehavior," "poor comportment," "bad conduct," and the like, in the form of getting out of one's seat, insubordination, throwing a spitball, sticking a pigtail in an inkwell, or even the rare breaking of a window seem like events of another era, events so mild in comparison to the aggression of today that it is hard to conceive them as the extremes of a shared continuum. Commenting on Westin's study of urban school violence for the years 1870 through 1950, Bayh (1975), observes: "If . . . the system has never been totally immune from incidents of student misbehavior, such problems have historically been viewed as a relatively minor concern seldom involving more than a few sporadic and isolated incidents" (p. 3). Rubel (1977) has correspondingly noted that fights between students have changed from skirmishes using words and fists to aggravated assaults with lethal weapons.

In a manner consistent with our interpretation of nonschool violence in Table 1.1, the years prior to the 1960s may appropriately be called the "preescalation period" in American school violence. Consistent with Bayh's observations, a 1956 National Education Association [NEA] survey reported that two-thirds of the 4,270 teachers sampled from across the United States reported that fewer than 1% of their students caused instances of disruption or disturbance, and "95 percent [of the responding teachers] described the boys and girls they taught as either exceptionally well behaved, or reasonably well behaved" (NEA, 1956, p. 17).

In 1975, the Bayh Senatorial Subcommittee issued its Safe School Report. This survey of 750 school districts indicated that in U.S. schools between 1970 and 1973, homicides increased by 18.5%, rapes and attempted rapes increased by 40.1%, robberies increased by 36.7%, assaults on students increased by 85.3%, assaults on teachers increased by 77.4%, burglaries in schools increased by 11.8%, drug and alcohol offenses increased by 37.5%, and the number of weapons confiscated by school personnel (pistols, knives, chunka sticks, and even sawed-off shotguns) increased by 54.4%. The National Association of School Security Directors (1975) reported that in 1974 there were 204,000 assaults and 9,000 rapes in American schools. Matters had gone a very long way from spitballs and pigtails. There were 18,000 assaults on teachers in 1955, 41,000 in 1971, and 63,000 in 1975; by 1979, the number of such attacks had risen to 110,000. The situation has not improved in the subsequent decade. In the 1988–1989 school year, compared to the preceding year, school crime increased 5% and in-school weapons possession rose 21% in California's public schools (Bureau of Justice Statistics, 1992). In a similar comparison, the New York City public school system reported a 35% increase in assaults on students and school staff, a 16% increase in harassment, a 24% increase in larceny, and an overall crime rate increase of 25%.

Note that the greatest increase in crime rate occurred at the elementary school level (Wetzel, 1989). The level of assaults on teachers in America's public schools is sufficiently high that the vocabulary of aggression has been expanded to include what Block (1977) called the "battered teacher syndrome": a combination of stress reactions including anxiety, depression, disturbed sleep, headaches, elevated blood pressure, and eating disorders. The National Center for Education Statistics (1992) reported in 1991 that nearly one out of five U.S. school teachers reported being verbally abused by students, 8% reported being physically threatened, and 2% indicated they had been attacked by students during the previous year.

The seriousness of these attacks on teachers notwithstanding, most aggression in America's schools is directed by students toward other students. Victimization data from 26 major American cities surveyed in 1974 and 1975 indicated that 78% of personal victimizations in schools (rapes, robberies, assaults, and larcenies) involved students (McDermott, 1979). Ban and Ciminillo (1977) report that in a national survey the percentages of principals who reported "unorganized fighting" between students had increased from 2.8% in 1961 to 18% in 1974. After examining much of the data on the correlates of aggression toward students, Ianni (1978) reports that seventh graders are most likely to be attacked, twelfth graders least likely; at about age 13 the risks of physical attack tend to be greatest. Fifty-eight percent of such attacks involve victims and offenders of the same race; 42% are interracial. It has also been demonstrated that the smaller the size of a minority group in a school, the more likely it is that its members will be victimized by members of other racial groups.

A 1990 report, aptly titled "Caught in the Crossfire," captures the central role of firearms in the more recent surge of school violence. From 1986 to 1990, 71 people (65 students and 6 employees) were killed by guns in American schools. Another 201 were seriously wounded, and 242 were held hostage at gunpoint. Older adolescents were most frequently perpetrators as well as victims. Such school gun violence grew from gang or drug disputes (18%), longstanding arguments (15%), romantic disagreements (12%), fights over possessions (10%), and accidents (13%). An estimated 270,000 students carry handguns to school one or more times each year. The American School Health Association (1989) estimates that 7% of boys and 2% of girls carry a knife to school every day.

The nature of leadership and governance in a school can be a major correlate of violence within its walls. A firm, fair, consistent principal leadership style, for example, has been shown to be associated with low levels of student aggression. Arbitrary leadership and severe disciplinary actions tend to characterize schools experiencing high levels of aggression. School size is a further correlate of school violence: The larger the school, the more likely its occurrence. Such a relationship may grow from the easier identification of students by other students in smaller schools, and such consequences of larger schools as nonparticipation in governance, impersonality, and crowding.

Crowding is a particularly salient school-violence correlate, as aggressive behavior occurs more frequently in the more crowded school locations—stairways, hallways, and cafeterias—and less frequently in

classrooms themselves. Other often-chronic casuality zones include lava-
tories, entrance and exit areas, and locker rooms. Student violence is
most likely to occur during the time between classes, and, for reasons
that may have to do with "spring-fever effects," during the month of
March. With a number of exceptions, school violence also correlates
with the size of the community in which the school is located. The
proportion of American schools reporting serious levels of aggressive
behavior is 15% in large cities, 6% in suburban areas, and 4% in rural
areas. Public school students were slightly more likely to be victimized
than were private school students.

AGGRESSION TOWARD PROPERTY

School vandalism, defined as acts that result in significant damage to
schools (Greenberg, 1969), has been characterized in terms of *perpetrator motivation* as predatory, vindictive, or wanton (Martin, 1961) and,
in terms of *perpetrator perception*, as acquisitive, tactical, ideological,
revengeful, playful, and malicious (Cohen, 1971). Across motivational
or perceptual subtypes, vandalism viewed collectively is an expensive
fact of American educational life. Although estimates for some years
have shown considerable variability, several reports indicate that, in
direct parallel to incidence statistics for aggression toward people in
schools, aggression toward property increased substantially in the several years ending in the mid-1970s, and then leveled off at an absolutely
high level (Casserly, Bass, & Garrett, 1980; Inciardi & Pottieger, 1978;
Rubel, 1977; New Jersey Commissioner's Report to the Education Committee, 1988; Wetzel, 1989). One hundred million dollars worth of
damage resulting from such school vandalism is reported to have occurred in 1969, $200 million in 1970, $260 million in 1973, $550 mil-
lion in 1975, and $600 million in 1977.[1] Matters have worsened in
subsequent years. Los Angeles County reported a 14-year vandalism
expenditure in its schools of $52 million due to property damage; $32
million was the result of arson, and $25 million was due to theft and
burglary of school property (California Department of Education, 1990).
In 1991, 11% of America's elementary school principals, and 14% of
its secondary school principals reported serious or moderate levels of
vandalism (National Center for Education Statistics, 1992).
    In 1977, 24,000 of America's 84,000 public schools reported the
occurrence of some major vandalism each month. Specifically, in those
84,000 schools, there were substantial numbers of reports each month
of trespassing (10.9%), breaking and entering (10%), theft of school
property (12.3%), property destruction (28.5%), fires or false alarms
(4.5%), and bomb threats (1.1%). In 1979, America's schools reported

20 million thefts and 400,000 acts of property destruction. By 1991, one of eight teachers and one of nine students in America's schools reported incidents of stealing within any given month (Miller & Prinz, 1991). Others report concurring data regarding continuing high levels of in-school theft (Harris, Gray, Rees-McGee, Carroll, & Zaremba, 1987; Hutton, 1985).

Arson, a particularly dangerous form of vandalism, deserves special comment. From 1950 to 1975, while the number of students in average daily attendance in American public schools was increasing by 86%, school arson increased 859% (Rubel, 1977). The annual cost of school fires increased from $17 million in 1950 to $106 million in 1975. Even discounting inflationary influences, the cost of school arson increased by 179% in constant dollars during this period. Arson levels in America's schools have continued to grow, in both incidences and dollar cost, in subsequent years (National Center for Education Statistics, 1992). Though window breaking is the most frequent single act of aggression toward property in schools, arson is clearly the most costly, typically accounting for approximately 40% of total vandalism costs annually.

Although early research suggested that most vandalism was committed by lower-class minority males (Bates, 1962; Clinard & Wade, 1958), acts of vandalism have since become distributed in a more egalitarian manner. The school vandal of today is just as likely to be white as nonwhite (Goldmeir, 1974), middle-class as lower-class (Howard, 1978), and (at least for graffiti and similar acts) female as male (Richards, 1976). Most vandals are 11 to 16 years old (Ellison, 1973); do not manifest more signs of disturbance on formal psychological evaluations than youngsters who do not vandalize (Richards, 1976); are frequently students who have been left back (Nowakowski, 1966); are often truant (Greenberg, 1974), and frequently have been suspended from school altogether (Yankelovich, 1975).

Greenberg (1969) reports that vandalism rates tend to be highest in schools with obsolete facilities and equipment and low staff morale. Leftwich (1977) found a similarly strong relationship between high teacher turnover rates and levels of vandalism. Mayer and Sulzer-Azaroff (1991), in their research on school "setting events" which appear to influence, or at least covary with, the occurrence of high levels of school vandalism, point to an overly punitive school environment, characterized in particular by (1) overuse of punitive control methods, (2) inadequate clarity of school and classroom rules and disciplinary policies, (3) inconsistent or weak administrative support and follow-through, and (4) inadequate attention and responsiveness to individual differences among students regarding academic matters and behavior management. In contrast, vandalism has been found to be unrelated to teacher–student ratios, to the proportion of minority students in the school, or

to the percentage of students whose parents were on welfare or unem-
ployed (Casserly et al., 1980). Also, community characteristics are also
often important influences upon in-school events. In this connection,
school vandalism tends to be correlated with community crime level,
geographic concentration of students, degree of nonstudent (intruder)
presence in school, and nature of family discipline.

It is instructive to note the factors associated with *low* levels of aggression toward property in schools. These include informal teacher–
teacher and teacher–principal interactions, high levels of teacher identification with the school, and low student dropout rates (Goldman,
1961). The Bayh (1975) Study also reported vandalism to be lower when
school rules were strictly but evenhandedly enforced, parents supported
strong disciplinary policies, students valued teachers' opinions of them,
teachers avoided the use of grades as disciplinary tools, and teachers
avoided the use of hostile or authoritarian behavior toward students.

In addition to those factors described thus far that may prove to
be causally related to aggression in schools, a large number of these
factors have already been proposed as just such antecedents. Aggression toward persons or property in schools has been held to result, in
part, from low student self-esteem, student frustration associated with
learning disabilities or emotional problems, insufficient student participation in school rule making, student exclusion, truancy, the
presence of intruders, gang influences, and student alcohol and drug
abuse. Also implicated have been an array of purported teacher inadequacies: disrespectfulness, callousness, disinterest, incompetence, and
middle-class bias. Schools themselves have been considered as well-
springs of violence and vandalism when they are too large, impersonal,
unresponsive, nonparticipatory, overregulated, oppressive, arbitrary,
or inconsistent. American society at large, less directly but perhaps more
basically, has been implicated as a multiple source of aggression in
schools. Widespread aggression outside of school, the breakdown of
the American family, television influences, ethnic conflict, unemployment, poverty, inadequate health services, and an array of related social ills have all been implicated.

After decades of what, at least in retrospect, seem like negligible
incidence rates, both classes of aggression increased precipitously during the late 1960s and early 1970s. The fact that they have plateaued
at very high levels since that time can give us little cause for comfort.
In fact, there are several reasons to suspect that these current data may
be serious underestimates. Inconsistent and imprecise definitions of
violence and vandalism, inaccurate or nonexistent record keeping, unwillingness to report acts of aggression, fear of reprisal, wider variance
in reporting procedures, and school administrator concern with appearing inadequate, each may lead to markedly underestimated and

underreported incidence statistics. In fact, it has been estimated that actual levels of school violence and vandalism may be as much as 50% higher than those generally reported (Ban & Ciminillo, 1977).

POTENTIAL SOLUTIONS

The response of the educational community to this immense and un-remitting problem has been energetic, creative, and sustained. A very large number of potential solutions have emerged, some aimed at students themselves, and others at teachers, administrators, or the wider community in which the school functions. The types of proposed solutions have been almost as varied as they are numerous; including humanistic, behavioral, electronic, architectural, organizational, curricular, administrative, legal approaches. Table 1.2 is a comprehensive presentation of these potential solutions to aggression in school, a presentation that provides both a sense of the sheer scope and number of such efforts, and a further introduction to the closer examination of several of the more promising of these solutions that follows. All of these interventions have in fact been implemented in one, and often in many, American schools. Some have been systematically evaluated for their impact on violence and vandalism; others have been examined more cursorily, and still others not at all.

Clearly, the magnitude and costs of school violence in the United States are substantial. Table 1.2 shows us that the response of the American education establishment to this painful and costly trend has been energetic, constructive, and, in the case of at least a few programs, demonstrably successful. Such initial success at controlling, reducing, or even preventing school violence may be enhanced considerably, we believe, when the techniques thus identified are not only refined and systematically implemented, but also when they are used in optimal combinations. This will be especially true, we feel, when these combinations of successful interventions are simultaneously targeted toward each of the sources immediately or implicitly responsible for school violence: the youngsters themselves, the teachers, the schools, and the larger community.

NOTE

1. As the NEA's (1977) report indicates, as these years passed and vandalism costs grew, approximately half of such costs were directly due to property damage incurred, and the remaining half represented indirect vandalism costs associated with hiring and supporting a security force, using security devices, and so forth. These total vandalism cost figures typically have not included one additional and major hidden cost of such property destruction: insurance.

TABLE 1.2. Attempted Solutions to School Violence and Vandalism

I. *Student oriented*
   Diagnostic learning centers
   Regional occupational centers
   Part-time programs
   Academic support services
   Group counseling
   Student advisory committee
   Student patrols (interracial)
   Behavior modification: Contingency management
                            Time-out
                            Response cost
                            Contracting
   Financial accountability
   School transfer
   Interpersonal skill training
   Problem-solving training
   Moral education
   Values clarification
   Individual counseling
   More achievable reward criteria
   Identification cards
   Peer counseling
   Participation in grievance resolution
   Security advisory council
   School safety committee

II. *Teacher oriented*
   Aggression-management training for teachers
   Increased teacher–student nonclass contact
   Teacher–student–administration group discussions
   Low teacher–pupil ratio
   Firm, fair, consistent teacher discipline
   Self-defense training
   Carrying of weapons by teachers
   Legalization of teacher use of force
   Compensation for aggression-related expenses
   Individualized teaching strategies
   Enhanced teacher knowledge of student ethnic milieu
   Increased teacher–parent interaction

III. *Curriculum*
   Art and music courses
   Law courses
   Police courses
   Courses dealing with practical aspects of adult life
   Prescriptively tailored course sequences
   Work–study programs
   Equivalency diplomas
   Schools with walls (partitioning)
   Schools within schools

(cont.)

TABLE 1.2 *(cont.)*

Learning centers (magnet schools, educational parks)
Continuation centers (street academies, evening high schools)
Minischools
Self-paced instruction
Idiographic grading

IV. *Administrative*
Use of skilled conflict negotiators
Twenty-four-hour custodial service
Clear lines of responsibility and authority among administrators
School safety committee
School administration–police coordination
Legal rights handbook
School procedures manual
Written codes of rights and responsibilities
Aggression-management training for administrators
Democratized school governance
Human relations courses
Effective intelligence network
Principal visibility and availability
Relaxation of arbitrary rules (regarding smoking, dressing, absences, etc.)

V. *Physical school alterations*
Installing extensive lighting
Blacking out all lighting
Reducing school size
Reducing class size
Closing off isolated areas
Increasing staff supervision
Speeding up repair of vandalism targets
Monitoring electronically for weapons detection
Making safety corridors (school to street)
Removing tempting targets for vandalism
Recessing fixtures where possible
Installing graffiti boards
Encouraging student-drawn murals
Painting lockers bright colors
Using ceramic-type, hard-surface paints
Sponsoring clean-up, pick-up, fix-up days
Paving or asphalting graveled parking areas
Using plexiglass or polycarbon windows
Installing decorative grillwork over windows
Marking all school property for identification
Using intruder detectors (microwave, ultrasonic, infrared, audio, video, mechanical)
Employing personal alarm systems
Altering isolated areas to draw foot traffic

VI. *Parent oriented*
Telephone campaigns to encourage PTA attendance
Antitruancy committee (parent, counselor, student)

(cont.)

TABLE 1.2 *(cont.)*

Parenting skills training
Parents as guest speakers
Parents as apprenticeship resources
Parents as work–study contacts
Increased parent legal responsibility for children's behavior
Family education centers

VII. *Security personnel*
Police–K-9 patrol units
Police helicopter surveillance
Use of security personnel for patrol
Crowd control
Intelligence gathering
Record keeping
Teaching (e.g., law)
Counseling
Home visits
Development of school security manuals

VIII. *Community oriented*
Helping-hand programs
Restitution programs
Adopt-a-school programs
Vandalism prevention education
Mass media publication of cost of vandalism
Open school to community use after hours
Improved school–juvenile court liaison
Family back-to-school week
Neighborhood Day
Vandalism watch on or near school grounds via mobile homes
Encouragement of reporting by CB users of observed vandalism
Community education programs
More and better programs for disruptive/disturbed youngsters

IX. *State and federal oriented*
Uniform violence and vandalism reporting system
State antiviolence advisory committee
Stronger gun-control legislation
Enhanced national moral leadership
Better coordination of relevant federal, state, community agencies
Stronger antitrespass legislaton
More prosocial child-labor laws

CHAPTER 2

Prevention

Although the control and reduction of student aggression is a main theme of this book (reflecting that emphasis in the real world of school aggression management), the *prevention* of such behavior is clearly preferable. To make prevention a viable possibility, researchers have sought to understand the causes and the correlates of child and adolescent aggression. While there has been some success in this regard, there has also been significant dissatisfaction with progress in education and psychology toward creating effective prevention-oriented interventions. However, early evidence seems to suggest that cognitive–behavioral approaches are especially promising for the development of preventive measures.

DEFINITION

Primary prevention of mental health difficulties refers to initiatives to improve the life situations of the masses of people such that mental health problems are made less likely to appear. Caplan (1964) described this primary level as well as secondary and tertiary prevention levels. Secondary prevention targets vulnerable or impaired individuals with help to either remove them from an at-risk status or improve their functioning to optimal levels. Tertiary prevention efforts are involved with people already quite impaired. Tertiary interventions are aimed at preventing further deterioration; improvement is not expected.

IMPLEMENTATION

Primary prevention interventions are targeted at groups that may or may not be known to be at-risk for particular dysfunctions. The interventions have a before-the-fact quality, that is, the programs are initiated before any problems are noted. Experience has shown that these primary prevention efforts must be built on solid research that establishes causal links to the specific behaviors to be prevented. Common-sense notions about what people need to be invulnerable to mental health problems have not always proved true. For example, the idea that people act rationally, that is, if given correct information they will make good decisions, has been a disappointingly incomplete understanding of human behavior (Chassin, Presson, & Sherman, 1985; Cowen, 1984).

Mounting primary prevention efforts has been difficult. By the 1970s the importance of lifestyle on physical health was widely recognized (7 out of 10 leading causes of death in the United States have critical behavioral determinants); however, the analogy to mental health was not widely accepted (Goldston, 1986; Heffernan & Albee, 1985). The Vermont Conferences on Primary Prevention (e.g., Albee & Joffe, 1977; Bond & Rosen, 1980; Forgays, 1978; Kent & Rolf, 1979) have provided consistent prods to mental health agencies and researchers to include preventive initiatives in their agendas. Although important and supportive research has been accomplished, a coordinated policy to both study and implement preventive interventions has been elusive (Goldston, 1986).

POTENTIAL TARGET LEVELS

Primary prevention programs aim at both reducing the possibility of dysfunction and at enhancing the quality of life. For example, when considering the options for primary prevention with children, Rosenberg and Reppucci (1985) identified four econological target levels with examples of known dysfunctional events. At the *individual level*, children are born with different temperaments and physical strengths and vulnerabilities. These differences make children likely to be well parented, easy to manage, and teachable. Children may suffer a history of abuse, parental rejection, or inappropriate expectations from their parents.

At the *familial level*, children may be a part of ineffective interactions among family members, conflictual spousal relationships, or they may emit behaviors that increase the probability of abuse from their parents. At the *community level*, children may experience isolation from helpful supports, family unemployment, and other types of unmanageable stress. And finally, at the *societal level*, children are embedded in cultures that may sanction physical punishment, be unsupportive of education, or uninvolved in facilitating family functioning.

These well-known stressors can be chosen as primary prevention targets as can activities that are competency enhancing. For example, teaching parenting skills and social problem solving, providing child development information, offering training in coping strategies useful in reducing and managing stress, and demonstrating ways of finding employment are additional possibilities for primary prevention programs that would likely deter the emergence of aggressive behavior.

Many programs are a combination of approaches. Preventing the abusive behavior of parents has become increasingly urgent; typical programs have made use of media campaigns, information dissemination, crisis lines, and referral services. In addition, more comprehensive programs have provided home visits by nurses for the first two years of a baby's life, some rooming-in of the baby with the new mother while still in the hospital, and the training of new parents in home safety, money management, use of leisure time, nutrition, and job location (Ayoub & Jacewitz, 1982; Gray, 1983; Gray, Cutler, Dean, & Kempe, 1976; Gray & Kaplan, 1980; Klaus & Kennell, 1976; Lutzker, Wesch, & Rice, 1984; Olds, 1984).

SCHOOL PROGRAMS

Child-Focused Versus Ecological

School-based prevention programs have been both child focused and more broadly ecologically based (Durlak, 1985). Examples of child-focused programs include affective education, social problem solving/coping skills, and prevention of academic problems (Baskin & Hess, 1980; Blechman, Kotanchick, & Taylor, 1981; Blechman, Taylor, & Schrader, 1981; Boike, 1986; Durlak, 1983; Hansford & Hattie, 1982; Jason, Durlak, & Holton-Walker, 1984; Medway & Smith, 1978; Rickel, Eshelman, & Loigman, 1983; Sharp, 1981).

Although the results of these child-focused interventions clearly challenge researchers to continue refinement, a meta-analysis of 40 primary prevention strategies indicates that approaches differ in their effectiveness (Baker, Swisher, Nadenichek, & Popowicz, 1984). The overall effect size of studies using the improvement of cognitive coping skills as the intervention was only about .26 (a small effect according to

Cohen, 1969). In contrast, communication skills training had an effect size of about 3.90 (.93 with outliers removed, a large effect). The overall effect size for primary prevention studies was about .55 (medium effect). This .55 effect size suggests that a person receiving primary preventive interventions whose score on a variable was that of the mean of the control group would improve on that variable .55 standard deviations above the mean. This would translate into a change from the 50th percentile on some hypothetical variable to the 73rd percentile.

Obviously, however, improvements vary according to the type of preventive intervention received. Career maturity enhancement, communication skills training, psychological education programs, and a combination of psychological and moral education programs all show large effect sizes, as do values clarification programs. Cognitive coping skills training programs, moral education programs (alone), substance abuse prevention programs, and programs blending values clarification with other strategies show low effect sizes (see Baker et al., 1984, for list of studies and specific effect sizes).

Ecological interventions with children in schools include classroom organization, interdependent learning, peer tutoring, parent programs, teacher programs, and program implementation research. These last three areas are badly neglected in terms of research, while the first three seem neglected by practitioners (Gump, 1980; Harris & Sherman, 1973; Jason, Frasure, & Ferone, 1981; Stallings, 1975).

Ecological interventions appear promising. For example, interventions involving interdependent learning or peer tutoring have been associated with improved attitudes toward school, better peer relations, and other social and academic gains for both tutors and tutees (Hightower & Avery, 1986). Classroom structures have been prescriptively described with open classrooms facilitating the achievement of high socioeconomic status and high-IQ students while worsening the achievement of low-IQ students. Increased structure has been associated with gains in math and reading, while less structure has facilitated growth in independence, cooperation, initiation, and reduced absenteeism. Overall, Stallings (1975) reports that about 40% of children's achievement can be accounted for by classroom instructional procedures and 30% by their entry abilities.

The earliest primary prevention program at the elementary school level, the St. Louis Project of 1947 (Glidewell, Gildea, & Kaufman, 1973), involved parents; however, more recent work at the elementary level has not included parents. This is in sharp contrast to preschool programs that have frequently and successfully included parental involvement (Gray & Wandersman, 1980; Lazar & Darlington, 1982).

Implementation realities have been overlooked and it is disheartening to consider that carefully conceptualized prevention programs may never be implemented correctly at classroom or building levels. Such may be the case, however, indicating a critical need to identify elements that affect the implementation process (Berman & McLaughlin, 1976; Fullan & Pomfret, 1977). Cowen (1980) summarizes both the promise and the problem of preventive intervention well with this observation:

> Primary prevention is a glittering, diffuse, thoroughly abstract term. Its aura is so exalted that some put it on the same plane as the Nobel Prize. It offers a sharp contrast to all that mental health has done, a shadowy, but nevertheless grand, alternative. It is terribly "major" in the lingo of childhood games I have known, something to be approached with massive giant steps. (p. 1)

Lorion (1983) cites the reality, however, that only small steps are possible given the developmental changes characteristic of children and the necessity to develop particular research bases for each intervention (i.e., generative base).

> In the absence of knowledge of a disorder's causes and/or of the individual, familial, and environmental conditions for its manifestations, the initiation of a primary prevention effort appears premature. Similarly, if ignorant of the preliminary manifestations of target disorders, unable to systematically detect their presence, or incapable of altering their evolution, one is unprepared to attach a problem at the secondary level. Finally, if we are unaware of how a specific skill develops and is maintained in the everyday environment, enhancement efforts may need to be deferred. (p. 265)

A critical analysis of prevention efforts will, therefore, suggest both hopeful beginnings of programs and strategies, and the enormity of the challenge. Preventing childhood problems *is* "terribly major," yet disquieting evidence of what is unknown or simply too expensive to implement is sobering.

School-Based Cognitive–Behavioral Prevention

Recent years have seen prevention programs and research both refine longstanding areas of interest and introduce new programs in response to societal pressures. The school has remained a favored environment in which to introduce prevention programs (Allen, Chinsky, Larsen, Lochman, & Selinger, 1976; Bower, 1965; Cowen, 1973, 1977, 1982, 1983;

Elias & Clabby, 1992). The advent of cognitive–behavioral approaches may be particularly attractive to school personnel because of the intuitive relationship between academic goals and those of cognitive training.

Social problem solving continues to attract attention, especially in terms of relating skills in problem solving or decision making to adjustment. Programs to combat student aggression, teenage pregnancy, substance abuse by children and youths, divorce support groups for children and parents, and programs to provide skills to children to avoid or report physical and sexual abuse are newer additions to the prevention armamentarium.

Each of the prevention approaches reviewed contains interventions reflecting core assertions of cognitive–behavioral therapy (Mahoney, 1977; Mahoney & Nezworski, 1985). These are:

1. Humans respond to cognitive representations of their environments rather than to the environments per se.
2. The cognitive representations are functionally related to the processes and parameters of learning.
3. Most human learning is cognitively mediated.
4. Thoughts, feelings, and behaviors are causally interactive.

A framework, commonly used in prevention research, may be a useful device to organize what is currently known or being attempted in the cognitive–behavioral area for prevention. When considering how children might avoid emotional, behavioral, learning, or adjustment problems, the challenge can be divided into interventions directed at the agent (those things or people that cause problems for children), environment (places where children spend their time and where they can experience either health-producing or debilitating effects), and host (the children themselves).

Social Problem Solving

Social problem solving (SPS) is the most mature of the cognitive–behavioral intervention approaches and is particularly attractive when considering the prevention of aggressive behavior. Based on Meichenbaum's (Asarnow & Meichenbaum, 1979; Meichenbaum & Burland, 1979; Meichenbaum & Goodman, 1969) pioneering work with impulsive children, SPS has attracted proponents primarily because of its promise as a "portable" reinforcement system. Efforts with SPS are aimed at hosts, that is, children themselves. Dismayed with the generalization problems so frequently encountered after apparently successful behavioral remediation, researchers and practitioners have seen SPS as a way for children to mediate their own behavioral programs and thus achieve social competence, that is, "those coordinated sets of behaviors that help people adapt effectively within the contexts of their social environment" (Kirschenbaum & Ordman, 1984, p. 381).

Certainly, behaviors that facilitate successful adaptation to the social environment are prime targets for prevention-minded professionals. Such adaptation, often called "adjustment" in the research literature, is the sine qua non of prevention. The consistent success of SPS training in improving the cognitive skills needed for dealing with analogue problems is an exciting finding. The inconsistency with which SPS is related to adjustment is a serious concern (Olsen & Work, 1986).

The most successful of the SPS training models, as related to prevention, is the work done by Spivack and Shure (1974; Bales, 1985; Pelligrini & Urbain, 1985). They have reported a decade of success in relating their teaching of interpersonal cognitive problem solving (ICPS) to teacher and parent appraisals of adjustment among trained children. The Spivack and Shure approach emphasizes alternative, consequential, and means–end thinking. In addition, children are taught social–cognitive competencies, for example, assertiveness, role taking, and familiarity with social rules and conventions. The combination of teaching social competencies as well as thinking skills, *in situ* contingently managed performance opportunities, and the simultaneous training of parents and teachers may be partially responsible for the uniquely successful work done by Shure and Spivack.

Other researchers (e.g., Elardo & Caldwell, 1979; Sharp, 1981; Urbain, 1980; Weissberg et al., 1981a, 1981b; Winer et al., 1982) who incorporated aspects of the ICPS models in their intervention programs, have had mixed and sometimes disconcerting results. Sharp and Weissberg et al.'s (1981b) findings that sometimes children's adjustment ratings declined while activity and aggressive behaviors increased following training are especially noteworthy.

Weissberg et al. (1981b) were able to isolate the effects of urban versus suburban environments in explaining their findings. Suburban children improved in both thinking skills and teacher ratings of adjustment. Urban children improved in thinking skills, but their adjustment ratings decreased. Urban teachers reported the brainstorming component of ICPS predictably led to aggressive, negative solutions and created discipline problems.

Weissberg et al.'s (1981a) revision of the program solved the discipline problems and the urban/suburban differences in adjustment ratings, but the adjustment ratings and thinking skills tests remained uncorrelated. That is, the children whose thinking skills improved were not necessarily those whose adjustment improved.

Elardo and Caldwell (1979), Durlak (1983), and Gesten et al. (1982) report more hopeful findings. Gesten's work may be especially informative to prevention researchers in that he found better results in children's adjustment and sociometric ratings a year after the completion of the program. Shure and Spivack (1979) reported similar findings and suggest that ICPS may inoculate young children against developing social adjustment problems.

Elias and Clabby (1992) have similarly reported on 12 years of promising research with their Improving Social Awareness–Social Problem Solving (ISA-SPS) model. Their recent book may have special appeal to practitioners because it outlines the realities of school policies that interact with setting up successful programs.

Rational Emotive Therapy

Ellis's rational emotive therapy (RET; Ellis, 1973; Ellis & Harper, 1975) and Maultsby's rational behavior therapy (RBT; 1971) are closely related to SPS and social skills training. Because RET and RBT are so similar, the following discussion uses RET to indicate both approaches.

RET's concern with the identification of self-defeating (irrational) thoughts, and conviction that people are disturbed more by their appraisals of events than by the events themselves, place it clearly within the province of cognitive–behavioral therapy. RET has been used extensively with youths of diverse types including aggressive children and adolescents (e.g., Beckmeyer, 1974; Bernard & Joyce, 1984; DiGiuseppe, 1975; Hauck, 1967; Knaus, 1974; Knaus & Boker, 1975; Maultsby, 1975; McMullin & Casey, 1974; Moleski & Tosi, 1976; Roush, 1984; Tosi, 1974; Young, 1974, 1975).

Of particular note has been the success of RET approaches in increasing grade-point averages and attendance, and decreasing disruptiveness and the discipline–referral–recidivism rates of high school students (Block, 1978; Warren, Smith, & Velten, 1984; Zelie, Stone, & Lehr, 1980). These variables are excellent markers of the successful adjustment of individuals to their school environments. RET in schools has been delivered via small counseling groups or as an alternative to the usual disciplinary response after a teacher referral. The use of RET in a group format increases its usefulness as a preventive intervention, as does the likelihood that RET could be incorporated into the usual procedures of a school program. RET has usually been offered to students on a weekly or twice-weekly basis for a class period over the course of 3 to 12 weeks (Cangelosi, Gressard, & Mines, 1980; Maultsby, Knipping, & Carpenter, 1974). Optimal time frames and intensities for RET training have not been well researched, but deserve attention, especially if large-scale prevention programs are envisioned.

Analysis

Several observations may be pertinent to the use of social problem solving and RET by professionals hoping to prevent aggressive behavior. First, most of the work in this area has focused on the host, that is the child, and has excluded considerations of the environment and the agent. Secondly, even this focus on the child has been narrow in that developmental considerations and other person variables (e.g., sex, ethnicity, preexisting skills, causal attributional style, motivation for change) have not been part of experimental designs. And finally, although there is evidence that time may be a factor in determining whether the generalized effects of training can be seen, most research still relies on brief posttesting periods with measures that may lack social validity.

These criticisms do not apply equally to all research. The ICPS work of Shure and Spivack (1979) and the ISA-SPS model of Elias and Clabby (1992) have both included training with teachers and parents. In this way, the child's environment has been changed and possible agent problems addressed. Spivack has identified the training of significant caregivers as the important difference between his and others' less successful work (Bales, 1985). In like manner, the application of RET in the schools has necessitated different adult responses to children's difficulties. Such adult changes may account for the success of the technique with children.

There is growing evidence that these techniques must be used prescriptively. For example, the experience of Weissberg et al. (1981a, 1981b) shows that social class may interact with the success of SPS programs. Olsen and Work (1986) suggest that children's empathy levels affect their success in applying SPS; those initially highest in empathy benefit most from training. Little is known about how developmental levels and basic cognitive processing strengths and deficits of the host interact with successful cognitive–behavioral interventions (Eastman & Rasbury, 1981). It seems obvious, however, that more effective training models could be established if these variables were taken into consideration. For example, because children's friendships change over time (e.g., from parallel play partner to confidante), the kinds of skills taught at different ages should be different (Kendall, 1985). In like manner, the severity of the problem being addressed, the host's preexisting skills and competencies, self-perceived efficacy, causal attribution for success and failure, motivation for change, and the quality of the child's school and home environments are all variables likely to contribute to treatment by subject interactions (Abikoff, 1985; Meichenbaum & Asarnow, 1979; Whalen, Henker, & Hinshaw, 1985).

Although attention to all these considerations is difficult under any circumstances, the need to individualize implies that SPS, social skills training, and even RET are not panaceas for preventive work. Mahoney and Nezworski (1985) categorize rationalistic versus developmental approaches in cognitive-behavior therapy, and their distinctions are valuable in the context of this discussion. They argue that teaching skills is probably not enough because the teaching must be done with a thorough knowledge of the inner person being taught. They assert that attention to the impact of early experience on individual differences in cognitive style, the role of affective processes in adaptation, the role of the family and other social systems on the acquisition of cognitive patterns, and the role of self-identity processes in psychological change and maintenance is crucial to the continued health of the cognitive–behavioral approaches to change.

The significant issues raised by Mahoney and Nezworski (1985) and others suggest that attention beyond the host is crucial. Well-trained teachers and parents could presumably accomplish the individualization of cognitive–behavioral programs that researchers find impossible to do because of internal validity concerns. The future of the SPS, social skills training, and RET as preventive interventions may depend on the application of the techniques to and by members of children's daily environments.

Despite mixed research findings, a broad analysis of what is currently extant in cognitive–behavioral therapy with such children does suggest an exciting future. Although no one strategy provides a perfect inoculation of children against future difficulties, combination approaches seem promising. Cognitive–behavioral techniques can be a part of a comprehensive prevention program that attends to hosts, environments, and agents.

PART II

STUDENT-ORIENTED INTERVENTIONS

CHAPTER 3

$+$

Psychological
Skills Training

Until the early 1970s, there were primarily three clusters of psychotherapies designed to alter the behavior of aggressive, unhappy, ineffective, or disturbed individuals: psychodynamic/psychoanalytic,
humanistic/client-centered, and behavior modification. Each of these
orientations found concrete expression in individual and group interventions targeted to aggressive adolescents and younger children. The
psychodynamic view was embodied in psychoanalytically oriented individual psychotherapy (Guttman, 1970), activity group therapy (Slavson, 1964), and the varied array of treatment procedures developed
by Redl and Wineman (1957). The humanistic/client-centered approach
was found in the applications to juvenile delinquents (e.g., Truax,
Wargo, & Silber, 1966) of the client-centered psychotherapy of Carl
Rogers (1957), the therapeutic community applications of Jones (1953),
guided group interaction (McCorkle, Elias, & Bixby, 1958), positive peer
culture (Vorrath & Brendtro, 1974), and the school discipline approach
of Dreikurs, Grunwald, and Pepper (1971). And behavior modification
was embodied in a wide variety of interventions reflecting the systematic
use of contingency management, contracting, and the training of
teachers and parents as behavior-change managers (O'Leary & Becker,
1967; Patterson, Cobb, & Ray, 1973; Walker, 1979).

Though each of these intervention philosophies differs from the
others in several major respects, one of their significant commonali-
ties is the shared assumption that the client is capable of performing
the effective, satisfying, nonaggressive, or prosocial behaviors whose

expression is among the goals of the intervention. Such latent poten-
tials would be realized by the client in all three approaches if the change
agent were sufficiently skilled in reducing or removing obstacles to such
realization. The psychodynamic therapist sought to do so by calling
forth and interpreting unconscious material blocking progress-relevant
awareness. The client-centered change agent, who, in particular, believed that the potential for change resides within the client, sought
to free this potential by providing a warm, empathic, maximally accepting helping environment. And the behavior modifier, by means of one
or more contingency management procedures, attempted to ensure that
when the latent desirable behaviors or approximations thereof did occur, the client would receive appropriate contingent reinforcement,
thus increasing the probability that these behaviors would recur. Therefore, whether sought by means of interpretation, therapeutic climate,
or contingent reward, all three approaches assumed that somewhere
within the individual's repertoire resided the desired, effective, sought-
after goal behaviors.

SKILL DEFICIENCY AND AGGRESSIVE YOUTH

A substantial body of literature has demonstrated that aggressive children and teenagers display a variety of interpersonal, planning, aggression management, and other psychological skill deficiencies. Freedman,
Rosenthal, Donahoe, Schlundt, and McFall (1978) examined the comparative skill competence levels of a group of juvenile delinquents and
a matched group (age, IQ, socioeconomic background) of nonoffenders
in response to a series of standardized role plays. The offender sample
responded in a consistently less skillful manner. Spence (1981) constitut-
ed comparable offender and nonoffender samples and videotaped interviews of each adolescent with a previously unknown adult. The
offender group showed significantly less eye contact, appropriate head
movement, and speech, and significantly more fiddling and gross body
movement. Conger, Miller, and Walsmith (1965) add further to this picture of skill deficiency. They conclude from their evidence that juvenile
delinquents, as compared to nondelinquent cohorts

> had more difficulty in getting along with peers, both in individual one-to-
> one contacts and in group situations, and were less willing or able to treat
> others courteously and tactfully, and less able to be fair in dealing with
> them. In return, they were less well liked and accepted by their peers. (p.
> 442)

Not only are delinquents discriminable from their nondelinquent peers on a continuum of skill competence, but much the same is true for youngsters who are "merely" chronically aggressive. Patterson, Reid, Jones, and Conger (1975) observe:

> The socialization process appears to be severely impeded for many aggressive youngsters. Their behavioral adjustments are often immature and they do not seem to have learned the key social skills necessary for initiating and maintaining positive social relationships with others. Peer groups often reject, avoid, and/or punish aggressive children, thereby excluding them from positive learning experiences with others. (p. 4)

ORIGINS OF PSYCHOLOGICAL SKILLS TRAINING

In the early 1970s, an important new intervention approach began to emerge: psychological skills training. This approach rested upon rather different assumptions. Viewing the person in need of help more in educational and pedagogical terms than in counseling or psychotherapeutic terms, the psychological skills trainer assumed such a person was lacking, deficient, or at best weak in the skills necessary for effective and satisfying personal and interpersonal functioning. The task of the skills trainer became, therefore, not interpretation, reflection, or reinforcement but the active and deliberate teaching of desirable behaviors. Rather than being like an intervention called psychotherapy that occurs between a patient and psychotherapist, or counseling between a client and a counselor, this intervention was a kind of training that took place between a trainee and a psychological skills trainer.

The roots of the psychological skills training movement lie in both education and psychology. The possibility of teaching desirable behaviors has often, if sporadically, been a significant goal of the American educational establishment. The character education movement of the 1920s and more contemporary moral education and values clarification programs are but a few of several possible examples. Add to this institutionalized educational interest in skills training the hundreds of interpersonal and planning skills courses taught in the more than 2,000 community colleges across the United States, and the hundreds of self-help books oriented toward similar skill-enhancement goals that are available to the public, and it becomes clear that the formal and informal educational establishment has provided fertile soil and explicit stimulation within which the psychological skills training movement could grow.

Much the same can be said for American psychology, as its prevailing philosophy and concrete interests have also laid the groundwork for the development of this new movement. The learning process has been the central theoretical and investigative concern of American psychology since the late 19th century, a concern that assumed major therapeutic form in the 1950s as psychotherapists and researchers alike came to view psychotherapeutic treatment more and more in learning terms. The very healthy and still expanding field of behavior modification grew from this joint learning–clinical focus, and may be viewed as the immediately preceding context from which psychological skills training emerged. Concurrent with the growth of behavior modification, psychological thinking increasingly shifted from a strict emphasis on remediation to one equally concerned with prevention, and the bases for this shift included movement away from a medical model concept toward a psychoeducational theoretical stance. Both of these movements—heightened concern with prevention and a psychoeducational perspective—gave impetus to the psychological skills training movement.

Perhaps psychology's most direct contribution to psychological skills training came from social learning theory and, in particular, from the work conducted or inspired by Albert Bandura. Regarding the same broad array of modeling, behavioral rehearsal, and social reinforcement investigations that helped stimulate and direct the development of our own approach to skills training, Bandura (1973) comments:

> The method that has yielded the most impressive results with diverse problems contains three major components. First, alternative modes of response are repeatedly modeled, preferably by several people who demonstrate how the new style of behavior can be used in dealing with a variety of ... situations. Second, learners are provided with necessary guidance and ample opportunities to practice the modeled behavior under favorable conditions until they perform it skillfully and spontaneously. The latter procedures are ideally suited for developing new social skills, but they are unlikely to be adopted unless they produce rewarding consequences. Arrangement of success experiences particularly for initial efforts at behaving differently, constitute the third component in this powerful composite method. ... Given adequate demonstration, guided practice, and success experiences, this method is almost certain to produce favorable results. (p. 253)

Other events of the 1970s provided still further stimulation for the growth of the skills training movement. The inadequacy of prompting, shaping, and related operant procedures for adding new behaviors to individuals' behavioral repertoires was increasingly apparent. The widespread reliance upon deinstitutionalization that lay at the heart of the community mental health movement resulted in the discharge of approximately 400,000 persons from public mental hospitals, the majority of whom were substantially deficient in important daily functioning skills. In addition, it had become clear that the American mental health movement had little to offer clients from the lower socioeconomic levels. These factors—relevant supportive research, the incompleteness of operant approaches, large populations of grossly skill-deficient individuals, and the paucity of useful interventions for large segments of American society—along with historically supportive roots in both education and psychology, suggested to several researchers and practitioners the need for a new intervention, something prescriptively responsive to the several deficiencies of existing interventions. Psychological skills training was the answer, and a movement was launched.

SKILLSTREAMING

A psychological skills training approach we have termed "skillstreaming" began in the early 1970s. At that time, and for several years thereafter, our studies were conducted in public mental health hospitals with long-term, highly skill-deficient, chronic patients, especially those preparing for deinstitutionalization into the community. As our research program progressed and regularly demonstrated successful skill-enhancement effects (Goldstein, 1981), we shifted our focus from teaching a broad array of interpersonal and daily living skills to adult psychiatric inpatients to a more explicit concern with skill training for aggressive individuals. Our trainee groups included spouses engaged in family disputes violent enough to warrant police intervention (Goldstein, Monti, Sardino, & Green, 1979; Goldstein & Rosenbaum, 1982), child-abusing parents (Goldstein, Keller, & Erne, 1985; Solomon, 1977; Sturm 1980), and most especially, overtly aggressive adolescents (Goldstein & Pentz, 1984; Goldstein, Sherman, Gershaw, Sprafkin, & Glick, 1978; Goldstein, Sprafkin, Gershaw, & Klein, 1980) and younger children (McGinnis & Goldstein, 1984).

IMPLEMENTATION OF PSYCHOLOGICAL
SKILLS TRAINING

Psychological skills training may be implemented via a variety of didactic procedures, but most such approaches revolve primarily around the four techniques that constitute skillstreaming: *modeling, role playing, per-*

formance feedback, and *transfer and maintenance of training.* After a brief overview of each, we will examine these procedures in greater detail.

Modeling

Skillstreaming requires first that trainees be exposed to good, clear examples of the behaviors (skills) we wish them to learn. The five or six trainees constituting the skillstreaming group are selected based upon their shared skill deficiencies. Each skill is broken down into four to six different behavioral steps that constitute the operational definition of the given skill. Using either live acting by the group's trainers or audiovisual modeling displays, actors portray the steps of that skill being used expertly in a variety of settings relevant to the trainee's daily life. Trainees are told to watch and listen closely to the way the actors in each vignette sequentially portray the skill's behavioral steps.

Role Playing

A brief spontaneous discussion almost invariably follows the presentation of a modeling display. Trainees frequently comment on the steps and the actors, and on how the problem portrayed occurs in their own lives. Since our primary goal in role playing is to encourage realistic behavioral rehearsal, a trainee's statements about difficulties using the skill being taught can often develop into material for the first role play. To enhance the realism of the portrayal, the main actor is asked to choose a second trainee (coactor) to play the role of a significant other person who is relevant to the skill problem.

The main actor is asked to describe briefly the real skill problem situation, and the person(s) involved with whom he or she could try the behavioral steps in real life. The coactor is called by the name of the main actor's significant other during the role play. The trainer then instructs the role players to begin. It is the trainer's responsibility at this point to be sure the main actor keeps role playing and that he or she attempts to follow the behavioral steps while doing so. Role playing is continued until all trainees in the group participate.

Performance Feedback

Upon completion of each role play, a brief feedback period ensues. The goals of this activity are (1) to let the main actor know how well he or she either followed the skill's steps or departed from them; (2) to explore the psychological impact of the enactment on the coactor, and to provide the main actor with encouragement to try out the role play behaviors in real life. Comments must point to the presence or absence of specific, concrete behaviors, and not take the form of general evaluative comments.

Transfer and Maintenance of Training

Several aspects of the skillstreaming sessions described above aim primarily to augment the likelihood that the learning that occurs in training will transfer to the trainee's real life environment and endure over time. These procedures include using: (1) general principles, (2) response availability, (3) identical elements, (4) stimulus variability, and (5) programmed reinforcement (Goldstein, 1981; Goldstein & Kanfer, 1979).

Coinciding with our development of the skillstreaming approach to psychological skills training, a number of similar programmatic attempts to enhance social competence have emerged. Those focusing at least to some extent on aggressive youngsters and their prosocial training include life skills education (Adkins, 1970), social skill training (Argyle, Trower & Bryant, 1974), AWARE: Activities for Social Development (Elardo & Cooper, 1977), relationship enhancement (Guerney, 1977), teaching conflict resolution (Hare, 1976), developing human potential (Hawley & Hawley, 1975), interpersonal communication (Heiman, 1973), and directive teaching (Stephens, 1976). The instructional techniques which constitute each of these skills training efforts derive from social learning theory and typically consist of instructions, modeling, role playing and performance feedback, with ancillary use in some instances of contingent reinforcement, prompting, shaping, or related behavioral techniques.

PREPARING FOR SKILLSTREAMING[1]

Selecting Trainers

A wide variety of individuals—their educational backgrounds ranging from high school diploma only through various graduate degrees—have served successfully as skillstreaming trainers. While formal training as a teacher or in a helping profession is both useful and relevant to becoming a competent skillstreaming trainer, we have found characteristics such as sensitivity, flexibility, and instructional talent to be considerably more important than formal education. We have made frequent and successful use of trainers best described as paraprofessionals, particularly with trainees from lower socioeconomic levels. In general, we select trainers based upon the nature and demands of the skillstreaming group.

Two types of trainer skills appear crucial for successfully conducting a skillstreaming group. The first might be described as general, that is, they are necessary for success in almost any training or teaching effort. These include (1) oral communication and teaching ability, (2) flexibility and resourcefulness, (3) enthusiasm, (4) ability to work under pressure, (5) interpersonal sensitivity, (6) listening skills, and (7) knowledge of their subject (child and adolescent development; aggression management; peer pressures on adolescents, etc.).

The second type are specific trainer skills, that is, those skills relevant to skillstreaming in particular. These include (1) knowledge of skillstreaming, its background, procedures, and goals; (2) ability to orient both trainees and supporting staff to skillstreaming; (3) ability to plan and present live modeling displays; (4) ability to initiate and sustain role playing; (5) ability to present material in concrete, behavioral form; (6) ability to deal with group management problems effectively; and (7) accuracy and sensitivity in providing corrective feedback.

How can we tell if potential trainers are skilled enough to become effective group leaders? We observe how competently potential trainers lead mock, and then actual, skillstreaming groups during our trainer preparation phase.

Preparing Trainers

We strongly believe in learning by doing. Our chief means of preparing trainers for skillstreaming group leadership is, first, to have them participate in an intensive, 2-day workshop designed to provide the knowledge and experience needed for a beginning competence. In the workshop, we use skillstreaming to teach skillstreaming. First, we assign relevant reading materials for background information. Next, trainees watch skilled group leaders demonstrate the modeling display presentation, the role playing, performance feedback, and the transfer training and maintenance procedures that constitute the core elements of the skillstreaming session. Then, workshop participants role play these group leadership behaviors in pairs and receive detailed feedback from the workshop leaders and others in the training group regarding the degree to which their group leadership behaviors matched or departed from those modeled by the workshop leaders. To help workshop learning transfer smoothly and fully to school or agency functioning, regular and continuing supervisory sessions are held after the workshop with the newly created skillstreaming group leaders. These booster/monitoring/supervision meetings, when added to the several opportunities available for trainer performance evaluation during the workshop itself, provide a large sample of behaviors on which to base a fair and appropriate trainer selection decision.

Selecting Trainees

Who belongs in the skillstreaming group? We have long held that no therapy or training approach is best for all clients and that our effectiveness as helpers or trainers will grow to a degree that we can become prescriptive in our helping efforts (Goldstein, 1978; Goldstein & Stein, 1976). As noted earlier, skillstreaming grew out of a behavior-deficit view of asocial and antisocial behavior. If such behavior is largely due to a lack of ability in a variety of prosocial skills of an interpersonal, personal, aggression management or related nature, our selection goal is defined for us. The skillstreaming group should consist of youngsters weak or deficient in one or more clusters of skills that constitute the skillstreaming curriculum. This selection process will involve optimally the use of interview, direct observation, behavioral testing procedures and appropriate skill checklists (Goldstein et al., 1980). Since the ultimate goals of skillstreaming are change in overt behavior, the removal of skill deficits, and the learning of prosocial alternatives, the selection of trainees focuses exclusively upon ascertaining the nature and level of skill deficiency.

Most of the usual bases for treatment or training selection are largely irrelevant to these selection decisions. If the clients are skill deficient and possess a few very basic group participation skills, we are unconcerned with their age, sex, race, social class, or, within very broad limits, even their mental health. At times we have had to exclude persons who were severely emotionally disturbed, too hyperactive for a 30-minute session, or so developmentally disabled that they lacked the rudimentary memory and imagery abilities necessary for adequate group participation. But such persons have been relatively few. Thus, while skillstreaming is not a prescription designed for all aggressive children and adolescents, its range of appropriate use is nevertheless quite broad.

Skillstreaming Skills

The 50 skills that constitute the skillstreaming curriculum for adolescents are listed below:

Group I. Beginning social skills
1. Listening
2. Starting a conversation
3. Having a conversation
4. Asking a question
5. Saying thank you
6. Introducing yourself
7. Introducing other people
8. Giving a compliment

Group II. Advanced social skills
9. Asking for help
10. Joining in
11. Giving instructions
12. Following instructions
13. Apologizing
14. Convincing others

Group III. Skills for dealing with feelings
15. Knowing your feelings
16. Expressing your feelings
17. Understanding the feelings of others
18. Dealing with someone else's anger
19. Expressing affection
20. Dealing with fear
21. Rewarding yourself

Group IV. Skill alternatives to aggression
22. Asking permission
23. Sharing something
24. Helping others
25. Negotiating
26. Using self-control
27. Standing up for your rights
28. Responding to teasing
29. Avoiding trouble with others
30. Keeping out of fights

Group V. Skills for dealing with stress
31. Making a complaint
32. Answering a complaint

33. Sportsmanship after the game
34. Dealing with embarrassment
35. Dealing with being left out
36. Standing up for a friend
37. Responding to persuasion
38. Responding to failure
39. Dealing with contradictory messages
40. Dealing with an accusation
41. Getting ready for a difficult conversation
42. Dealing with group pressure

Group VI. Planning skills
43. Deciding on something to do
44. Deciding what caused a problem
45. Setting a goal
46. Deciding on your abilities
47. Gathering information
48. Arranging problems by importance
49. Making a decision
50. Concentrating on a task

Each of the 50 skills is broken down into its constituent behavioral steps. The steps *are* the skill, and as such form the specific basis and guide for the entire modeling, role playing, performance feedback, transfer and maintenance sequence.

Group Organization

The preparation phase of the skillstreaming group is completed by attention to those organizational details necessary for a smoothly initiated, appropriately paced, and highly instructional group to begin. Factors to be considered in organizing the group are number of trainees, number of trainers, number of sessions, and spacing of sessions.

Number of Participants

Trainees

Since trainee behavior in a skillstreaming group may vary greatly, we cannot recommend a single, specific number of trainees as optimal. Ideally, the number of trainees will permit everyone to role play, will lead to optimal levels of group interaction, and will provide a diverse source of performance feedback opportunities. In our experience with aggressive children and adolescents, these goals have usually been met when the group's size was five to seven trainees.

Trainers

The role playing and feedback that make up most of each skillstreaming session are a series of action–reaction sequences in which effective skill behaviors are first rehearsed (role played) and then critiqued (feedback) in the context of a group not infrequently displaying behavior management problems. Thus, the trainer must lead, observe, and manage. We have found that one trainer is hard pressed to do these tasks all at the same time, and we strongly recommend that each session be led by a team of two trainers. One trainer can usually pay special attention to the main actor, helping the actor "set the stage" and enact the skill's behavioral steps. While this is occurring, the other trainer can attend to the remainder of the group and help them as they observe and evaluate the unfolding role play. The two trainers can then exchange these responsibilities on the next role play.

Sessions

Number

Skillstreaming groups typically seek to cover one skill in one or two sessions. The central task is to make certain that every trainee in the group role plays the given skill correctly at least once, preferably more than once. Most skillstreaming groups have met this curriculum requirement by holding sessions once or twice per week. Groups have varied greatly in the total number of meetings they have held.

Spacing

The goal of skillstreaming is not merely skill learning or acquisition; much more important is skill transfer. Performance of the skill in the training setting is desired, but performance of it in the school or community is crucial. Several aspects of skillstreaming are designed to enhance the likelihood of such skill transfer; session spacing is one such factor. As we will describe later, after the trainee role plays successfully in the group and receives thorough performance feedback, he or she is assigned homework, that is, the task of carrying out in the real world the skill just performed correctly in the group. In order to ensure ample time and opportunity to carry out this important task, skillstreaming sessions must be scheduled at least a few days apart.

Length and Location

One-hour sessions are the typical skillstreaming format, though both somewhat briefer and somewhat longer sessions have been successful. In general, the session goal that must be met is successful role playing and clarifying feedback for all participants, be it in 45 minutes, 1 hour, or 1 ½ hours.

In most schools, a reasonably quiet and comfortable office, classroom, or similar setting can be found or created for the use of skillstreaming groups. We suggest only that the meeting place be free of distraction, be minimally equipped with chairs and chalkboard, and have adequate lighting. How should the room be arranged? Again, no fixed pattern is required, but one functional and comfortable layout is the horseshoe or U-shaped arrangement, with the role players and the trainer guiding them at the front of the room. In this group arrangement, all observing trainees and the main actor can watch the trainer point to the given skills' behavioral steps written on the chalkboard while the role play is taking place. In this manner, any necessary prompting is provided immediately, and at the same time the role play is serving as an additional modeling display for the trainees.

Meeting with the Trainees Before the First Session

A final step that must be taken before holding the first session of a new skillstreaming group is preparing the new trainees for what to expect and what will be expected of them. This premeeting might include the following:

1. *Describing what the purposes of the group will be as they relate to the trainee's specific skill deficits.* For example, the trainer might say, "Remember when you were given in-school suspension because you thought Henry had insulted you and you got in a shoving match with him? Well in skillstreaming you'll be able to learn what to do in a situation like that so you can handle it without fighting and still settle calmly whatever is going on."

2. *Describing briefly the procedure that will be used.* While we believe that trainees typically will not have a full understanding of what skillstreaming is and what it can accomplish until after the group has begun, verbal, pregroup structuring of procedures is a useful beginning. It conveys at least a part of the information necessary to help trainees know what to expect. The trainer might say, "In order to learn to handle these problem situations better, we're going to see and hear some

examples of how different people handle them well. Then you will actually take turns trying some of these ways right here. We'll let you know how you did, and you'll have a chance to practice on your own."

3. *Describing the benefits of active trainee participation in the group.* If the trainer has relevant information from a trainee, the possible benefits described might include improved proficiency in the particular skillstreaming skills in which the trainee feels especially deficient.

4. *Describing group rules.* These include whatever rules the trainer believes the group members must adhere to in order to function smoothly and effectively with regard to attendance, punctuality, confidentiality, completion of homework assignments, and so forth. At this premeeting stage, rule structuring should be brief and tentative. Reserve a fuller discussion of this matter for the group's first session, in which all members can be encouraged to participate and in which rule changes can be made by consensus.

CONDUCTING THE SKILLSTREAMING GROUP

The Opening Session

The opening session is designed to create a safe, nonthreatening environment for trainees, stimulate their interest in the group, and give more detailed information about skillstreaming than was provided initially. The trainers open with a brief familiarization period of warmup to help participants become comfortable when interacting with the group leaders and with one another. Content for this initial phase should be interesting and nonthreatening to the trainees. Next, trainers introduce the skillstreaming program by providing trainees with a brief description of what skill training is about. Typically, this introduction covers such topics as the importance of interpersonal skills for effective and satisfying living, examples of skills that will be taught, and how these skills can be useful to trainees in their everyday lives. It is often helpful to expand this discussion of everyday skill use to emphasize the importance of the undertaking and the relevance that learning the skill can have to the participants. The specific training procedures (modeling, role playing, performance feedback, and transfer and maintenance training) are then described at a level that the group can easily understand. We recommend that trainers describe procedures briefly, with the expectation that trainees will understand them more fully once they have actually participated in their use. A detailed outline of the procedures that ideally make up this opening session follows.

Outline of Opening Session Procedures

A. Introductions.
   1. Trainers introduce themselves.
   2. Trainers invite trainees to introduce themselves if they are not all previously acquainted. As a way of relaxing trainees and beginning to familiarize them with one another, the trainer can elicit from each trainee some nonprivate information such as neighborhood of residence, school background, special interests or hobbies, and so forth.

B. Overview of skillstreaming.
Although some or all of this material may have been discussed in earlier individual meetings with trainees, a portion of the opening session should be devoted to a presentation and group discussion of the purposes, procedures, and potential benefits of skillstreaming. The discussion of the group's purposes should stress the probable remediation of those skill deficits that trainees in the group are aware of, concerned about, and eager to change. The procedures that make up the typical skillstreaming session should be explained again and discussed with give and take from the group. The language used to explain the procedures should be geared to the trainees' level of understanding, that is, "show," "try," "discuss," and "practice," respectively, for the words "modeling," "role playing," "performance feedback," and "transfer training." Perhaps heaviest stress at this point should be placed on presenting and examining the potential benefits to trainees of their participation. Concrete examples of the diverse ways that skill proficiencies can have a positive effect on the lives of trainees should be the focus of this effort.

C. Group rules.
The rules that will govern participation in the skillstreaming group should be presented by the trainers during the opening session. If appropriate, this presentation should permit and encourage group discussion designed to give members a sense of participation in the group's decision making. That is, members should be encouraged to accept and live by those rules they agree with and seek to alter those they wish to change. Group rules may be necessary and appropriate concerning attendance, lateness, size of the group, and time and place of the meetings. This is also a good time to provide reassurance to group members about concerns they may have, such as confidentiality, embarrassment, and fear of performing.

    Following introductions, the overview of skillstreaming, and the presentation of group rules, the trainers should introduce and model the group's first skill, conducting role plays on that skill, giving performance feedback, and encouraging transfer training. These activities make up all subsequent skillstreaming sessions.

Modeling

The modeling display presented to trainees should depict the behavioral steps that constitute the skill being taught in a clear and unambiguous manner. All of the steps making up the skill should be modeled in their correct sequence. Generally, the modeling will consist of live vignettes enacted by the two trainers. When two trainers are not available, a reasonably skillful trainee may serve as a model along with the trainer. In all instances, it is especially important to rehearse the vignettes carefully prior to the group meeting, making sure that all of the skill's steps are enacted correctly and in proper sequence.

Trainers should plan their modeling display carefully. Content should be selected that is relevant to the immediate life situations of the trainees in the group. At least two examples should be modeled for each skill so that trainees are exposed to skill use in different situations. Thus, two or more different content areas are depicted. We have found that trainers usually do not have to write out scripts for the modeling display but can instead plan their roles and likely responses in outline form and rehearse them in their preclass preparations. These outlines should incorporate the guidelines that follow:

1. Use at least two examples of different situations for each demonstration of a skill. If a given skill is taught in more than one group meeting, develop two more new modeling displays.
2. Select situations that are relevant to the trainees' real life circumstances.
3. The main actor, that is, the person enacting the behavioral steps of the skill, should be portrayed as a person reasonably similar in age, socioeconomic background, verbal ability, and other salient characteristics to the people in the skillstreaming group.
4. Modeling displays should depict only one skill at a time. All extraneous content should be eliminated.
5. All modeling displays should depict all the behavioral steps of the skill being modeled in the correct sequence.
6. All displays should depict positive outcomes. Displays should always end with reinforcement to the model.

In order to help trainees attend to the skill enactments, skill cards, which contain the name of the skill being taught and its behavioral steps, are distributed prior to the modeling display. Trainees are told to watch and listen closely as the models portray the skill. Particular care should be given to helping trainees identify the behavioral steps as they are presented in the context of the modeling vignettes. Trainers should also remind the trainees that in order to depict some of the behavioral steps in certain skills, the actors will occasionally be "thinking out loud" statements that would ordinarily be thought silently, and that this process is done to facilitate learning.

Role Playing

Following the modeling display, discussion should focus on relating the modeled skill to the lives of trainees. Trainers should invite comments on the behavioral steps and how these steps might be useful in real life situations. It is helpful to focus on current and future skill use rather than only on past events or general issues involving the skill. Role playing in skillstreaming is intended to serve as behavioral rehearsal or practice for future use of the skill. Role playing of past events that have little relevance for future situations is of limited value to trainees. However, discussion of past events involving skill use can be relevant in stimulating trainees to think of times when a similar situation might occur in the future. The hypothetical future situation, rather than a reenactment of the past event, would be selected for role playing.

Once a trainee has described a situation in his or her own life in which the skill might be helpful, that trainee is designated the main actor and is asked to choose a second trainee (the coactor) to play the role of the other person (mother, peer, staff member, etc.) who is relevant to the situation. The trainee should be urged to pick as a coactor someone who resembles the real life person in as many ways as possible — physically, expressively, and so on. The trainers then elicit from the main actor any additional information needed to set the stage for role playing. To make role playing as realistic as possible, the trainers should obtain a description of the physical setting, a description of the events immediately preceding the role play, a description of the manner the coactor should display, and any other information that would increase realism.

It is crucial that the main actor use the behavioral steps that have been modeled. This is the main purpose of the role playing. Before beginning to role play, the trainer should go over each step as it applies to the particular role play involved, thus preparing the main actor to make a successful effort. The main actor is told to refer to the skill card on which the behavioral steps are printed. As noted previously, the behavioral steps are written on a chalkboard visible to the main actor as well as the rest of the group during the role playing. Before the role playing begins, trainers should remind all of the participants of their roles and responsibilities. The main actor should be told to follow the behavioral steps, the coactor to stay in the role of the other person, and the observers to watch carefully for the enactment of the behavioral steps. At times, feedback from other trainees is facilitated by assigning each one a single behavioral step to focus upon and provide feedback about after the role play. For the first several role plays, the observers also can be coached on the kinds of cues (posture, tone of voice, content of speech, etc.) to observe.

During the role play, one of the trainers should provide the main actor with whatever help, coaching, and encouragement is needed to keep the role playing going according to the behavioral steps. Trainers who "break role" and begin to explain their behavior or make observer-like comments should be urged to get back into the role and explain later. If the role play is clearly going astray from the behavioral steps, the scene can be stopped, instruction can be provided, and then the role play can be restarted. One trainer should be positioned near the chalkboard in order to point to each of the behavioral steps in turn as the role play unfolds, thus helping the main actor (as well as the other trainees) to follow each of the steps in order. The second trainer should sit with the observing trainees to be available as needed to keep them on task.

The role playing should continue until all trainees have had an opportunity to participate in the role of main actor. Sometimes this will require two or three sessions for a given skill. As we suggested before, each session should begin with two new modeling vignettes for the chosen skill, even if the skill is not new to the group. It is important to note once again that while the framework (behavioral steps) of each role play in the series remains the same, the actual content can and should change from role play to role play. It is the problem as it actually occurs, or could occur, in each trainee's real life environment that should be the subject of the given role play.

There are other ways to increase the effectiveness of role playing. Role reversal is often a useful role play procedure. A trainee role playing a skill may on occasion have a difficult time perceiving the coactor's viewpoint and vice versa. Having them exchange roles and resume the role play can be most helpful in this regard. At times, the trainer can also assume the coactor role in an effort to give the trainee the opportunity to handle types of reactions not otherwise role played during the session. For example, it may be crucial to have a difficult coactor realistically portrayed. The trainer as coactor may also be particularly helpful when dealing with less verbal or more hesitant trainees.

Performance Feedback

A brief feedback period follows each role play. This helps the main actor find out how well he or she followed or departed from the behavioral steps. It also examines the psychological impact of the enactment on the coactor and provides the main actor with encouragement to try out the role played behaviors in real life. The trainer should ask the main actor to wait until everyone's comments have been heard before responding to any of them.

The coactor is asked about his or her reactions first. Next the observers comment on how well the behavioral steps were followed and about other relevant aspects of the role play. Then the trainers comment on how well the behavioral steps were followed and provide social reinforcement (praise, approval, encouragement) for close following. To be most effective in their use of reinforcement, trainers should follow these guidelines:

1. Provide reinforcement only after role plays that follow the behavioral steps.
2. Provide reinforcement at the earliest appropriate opportunity after role plays that follow the behavioral steps.
3. Vary the specific content of the reinforcements offered, for example, praise particular aspects of the performance, such as tone of voice, posture, phrasing, and so forth.
4. Provide enough role playing activity for each group member to have sufficient opportunity to be reinforced.
5. Provide reinforcement in an amount consistent with the quality of the given role play.
6. Provide no reinforcement when the role play departs significantly from the behavioral steps (except for "trying" in the first session or two).
7. Provide reinforcement for an individual trainee's improvement over previous performances.
8. Always provide reinforcement to the coactor for being helpful, cooperative, and so on.

In all aspects of feedback, it is crucial that the trainer maintain the behavioral focus of skillstreaming. Both trainers' and trainees' comments should point to the presence or absence of specific, concrete behaviors and not take the form of broad generalities. Feedback, of course, may be positive or negative in content. Negative comments should always be followed by a constructive comment as to how a particular fault might be improved. A "poor" performance can be praised as "a good try" at the same time it is being criticized for its real faults. If at all possible, trainees failing to follow the behavioral steps in their role play should be given the opportunity to repeat their performance after receiving corrective feedback. At times, as a further feedback procedure, we have audio- or videotaped entire role plays. Giving trainees post-role-play opportunities to observe themselves on tape can be an effective aid, enabling them to reflect on their own verbal and nonverbal behavior and its impact upon others.

Since a primary goal of skillstreaming is skill flexibility, role play enactments that depart somewhat from the behavioral steps may not be wrong, that is, a different approach to the skill may work in some situations. Trainers should stress that they are trying to teach effective alternatives and that the trainees would do well to have the behavioral steps being taught, or as collaboratively modified, in their repertoire of skill behaviors.

Transfer and Maintenance Training

Several aspects of the training sessions already described have been designed primarily to make it likely that learning in the training setting will transfer to the trainees' real life environments, and maintain there. Techniques for enhancing transfer and maintenance as they are used in the sessions follow.

Providing General Principles

It has been demonstrated that transfer and maintenance of training is facilitated by providing trainees with general mediating principles governing successful or competent performance in both the training and applied real world settings. This has been operationalized by providing subjects with the organizing concepts, principles, strategies, or rationales that explain the stimulus–response relationships operating in both the training and application settings. General principles of skill selection and utilization are provided to trainees verbally, visually, and in written form.

Overlearning

Overlearning involves training in a skill beyond what is necessary to produce initial changes in behavior. The overlearning, or repetition of successful skill enactment, in the typical skillstreaming session is quite substantial. Each skill is (1) modeled several times; (2) role played one or more times by the trainee; (3) observed by the trainee as every other group member role plays; (4) read by the trainee from a chalkboard and a Skill Card; and (5) practiced in real life settings one or more times by the trainee as part of a formal homework assignment.

Identical Elements

In perhaps the earliest research on transfer enhancement, Thorndike and Woodworth (1901) concluded that when one habit facilitated another, it was to the extent that they shared identical elements. More recently, Ellis (1965) and Osgood (1953) have emphasized the importance for transfer of similarity between the stimulus used in training and in application tasks. The greater the similarity between physical and interpersonal stimuli in the skillstreaming setting and the setting in which the skill is to be applied, the greater the likelihood of transfer. Skillstreaming is made similar to real life in several ways. These include

1. Designing the live modeling displays to be highly similar to what trainees face in their daily lives through the representative, relevant, and realistic portrayal of the models, protagonists, and situations.
2. Making the physical arrangement of the setting, and the co-actors as realistic as possible.
3. Conducting the role plays so they are as responsive as possible to the real life interpersonal stimuli to which trainees must respond later with the given skill.
4. Rehearsing each skill in role plays as the trainees actually plan to use it.
5. Assigning work to be done at home.

Stimulus Variability

Positive transfer is more likely when a variety of relevant training stimuli are employed (Callantine & Warren, 1955; Duncan, 1958; Shore & Sechrest, 1961). Stimulus variability may be implemented in skillstreaming sessions by

1. Rotating group leaders across groups.
2. Rotating trainees across groups.
3. Letting the role play of a given skill be done by trainees with several different coactors.
4. Role playing a given skill in several settings.
5. Completing multiple homework assignments for each given skill.

Real Life Reinforcement

Even with the successful implementation of both appropriate skill-streaming procedures and transfer and maintenance enhancement procedures, positive transfer and maintenance may still fail to occur. As Agras (1967), Gruber (1971), Patterson and Anderson (1964), Tharp and Wetzel (1969), and dozens of other more recent investigators have shown, stable and enduring performance in application settings of newly learned skills is very much at the mercy of real life reinforcement contingencies. We have found it useful to implement several supplemental programs outside of the skillstreaming setting that can help to provide the rewards trainees need in order to maintain new behaviors. These programs include provision for both external social rewards (provided by people in the trainee's real life environments) and self-rewards (provided by the trainees themselves). A particularly useful tool for transfer and maintenance enhancement, a tool combining the possibilities of identical elements, stimulus variability, and real life reinforcement, is the skill homework assignment.

In this procedure, trainees are instructed to try the behaviors they have practiced during the session in their own real life settings. The name of the person(s) with whom they will try the skill, the day, the place, and the like are all discussed. The trainee is urged to take notes on any attempt to use the skill, on the Homework Report form (Figure 3.1). This form requests detailed information from the trainee about what happened when the homework assignment was attempted and how well the relevant behavioral steps were followed. The trainee is asked to evaluate his or her performance, and to express any thoughts about what the next assignment might appropriately be.

It has often been useful to start with relatively simple homework behaviors and, as mastery is achieved, work up to more complex and demanding assignments. This provides both the trainer and the people who are targets of the homework with an opportunity to reinforce each approximation of the more complex target behavior. Successful experiences at beginning homework attempts are crucial in encouraging the trainee to make further attempts at real life use of the skill.

The first part of each skillstreaming session is devoted to presenting and discussing these homework reports. When trainees have made an effort to complete their homework assignments, trainers should provide social reinforcement, while failure to do homework should be met with some chagrin and expressed disappointment, followed by support and encouragement to complete the assignment. Without these or similar attempts to maximize transfer, the value of the entire training effort is in severe jeopardy.

Name _____ Date_____

Group leaders _____

Fill in during this class
1. Homework assignment:
   a. Skill:
   b. Use with whom:
   c. Use when:
   d. Use where:
2. Steps to be followed:

Fill in before next class
3. Describe what happened when you did the homework assignment:

4. Steps you actually followed:

5. Rate yourself on how well you used the skill (check one):

   Excellent_____ Good_____Fair_____Poor_____
6. Describe what you feel should be your next homework assignment:

FIGURE 3.1. Homework Report form.

Outline of Subsequent Session Procedures

A. Homework review.
B. Trainer presents overview of the skill.
  1. Introduces skill briefly prior to showing modeling display.
  2. Asks questions that will help trainees define the skill in their own language.
     Examples: "Who knows what _____ is?"; "What does _____ mean to you?"; "Who can define _____?"
  3. Postpones lengthier discussion until after trainees view the modeling display. If trainees want to engage in further discussion, the trainer might say, "Let's wait until after we've seen some examples of people using the skill before we talk about it in more detail."
  4. Makes a statement about what will follow the modeling display. Example: "After we see the examples, we will talk about times when you've had to use _____ and times when you may have to use that skill in the future."
  5. Distributes skill cards, asking a trainee to read the behavioral steps aloud.

6. Asks trainees to follow each step in the modeling display as the step is depicted.
C. Trainer presents modeling display.
1. Provides two relevant examples of the skill in use, following its behavioral steps.
D. Trainer invites discussion of skill that has been modeled.
1. Invites comments on how the situation modeled may remind trainees of situations involving skill usage in their own lives.
Example: "Did any of the situations you just saw remind you of times when you have had to _____?"
2. Asks questions that encourage trainees to talk about skill usage and problems involving skill usage.
Examples: "What do you do in situations where you have to _____?"; "Have you ever had to _____?"; "Have you ever had difficulty _____?"
E. Trainer organizes role play.
1. Asks a trainee who has volunteered a situation to elaborate on his or her remarks, obtaining details on where, when, and with whom the skill might be useful in the future.
2. Designates this trainee as a main actor, and asks the trainee to choose a coactor (someone who reminds the main actor of the person with whom the skill will be used in the real life situation).
Examples: "What does _____ look like?"; "Who in the group reminds you of _____ in some way?"
3. Gets additional information from the main actor, if necessary, and sets the stage for the role playing (including props, furniture arrangement, etc.).
Examples: "Where might you be talking to _____?"; "How is the room furnished?"; "Would you be standing or sitting?"; "What time of day will it be?"
4. Rehearses with the main actor what to say and do during the role play.
Examples: "What will you say for step one of the skill?"; "What will you do if the coactor does _____?"
5. Gives each group member some final instructions about what to say and do just prior to role playing.
Examples: To the main actor: "Try to follow all of the steps as best you can." To the coactor: "Try to play the part of _____ as best you can. Say and do what you think _____ would do when _____ follows the skill's steps." To the other trainees in the group: "Watch how well _____ follows the steps so that we can talk about it after the role play."

F. Trainer instructs the role players to begin.
   1. One trainer stands at the chalkboard and points to each step as it is enacted and provides whatever coaching or prompting is needed by the main actor or coactor.
   2. The other trainer sits with the observing trainees to help keep them attending to the unfolding role play.
   3. In the event that the role play strays markedly from the behavioral steps, the trainers stop the scene, provide needed instruction, and begin again.
G. Trainer invites feedback following role play.
   1. Asks the main actor to wait until everyone has had a chance to comment before talking.
   2. Asks the coactor, "In the role of _____, how did _____ make you feel? What were your reactions?"
   3. Asks observing trainees: "How well were the behavioral steps followed?" "What specific things did you like or dislike?" "In what ways did the coactor do a good job?"
   4. Comments on the following of the behavioral steps, provides social reward, points out what was done well, and comments on what else might be done to make the enactment even better.
   5. Asks main actor: "Now that you have heard everyone's comments, how do you feel about the job you did?" "How do you think that following the steps worked out?"
H. Trainer helps role player to plan homework.
   1. Asks the main actor how, when, and with whom he or she might attempt the behavioral steps prior to the next class meeting.
   2. As appropriate, the Homework Report form may be used to get a written commitment from the main actor to try out the new skill and report back to the group at the next meeting.
   3. Trainees who have not yet had a chance to role play may also be assigned homework in the form of looking for situations relevant to the skill that they might role play during the next class meeting.

MANAGING PROBLEM BEHAVIORS IN THE SKILLSTREAMING GROUP

As is true for any type of treatment, training, or teaching group, management problems sometimes occur during skillstreaming. Problems include any behaviors shown by one or more group members that interfere with, inhibit, deflect, or slow down the skills training procedures or goals that are the basic purposes of skillstreaming. Such behaviors are sometimes displayed by chronically aggressive children and adolescents, as they enact within the skillstreaming group the very behaviors which initially made their inclusion in the group appropriate. Some occur rarely, others with somewhat greater frequency.

Our coverage should be considered comprehensive but not exhaustive, since every time we have concluded that we've seen everything in the skillstreaming group, something new and challenging comes along. Our proposals for dealing with group management problems will usually suffice, but skilled trainers will be needed occasionally to deal creatively and imaginatively with new challenges as they arise, even in the most productive skillstreaming groups. Most methods for reducing problems will only be necessary to bridge initial trainee resistance and later trainee acceptance, when the trainee feels skillstreaming participation to be useful, valuable, and personally relevant. These techniques, derived from research on skills training group management as well as from our own experiences and those of others with such groups, should help trainers deal with almost any difficulties that may arise in the skillstreaming group.

Types of Group Management Problems

Inactivity

Minimal Participation. Minimal participation involves trainees who seldom volunteer, provide only brief answers, and in general give the trainers a feeling that they are "pulling teeth" to keep the group at its various skills training tasks.

Apathy. A more extreme form of minimal participation is apathy, when whatever the trainers do to direct, enliven, or activate the group is met with disinterest, lack of spontaneity, and little, if any, progress toward group goals.

Falling Asleep. While it is rare, trainees do fall asleep from time to time. The sleepers should be awakened, and the trainers might wisely inquire into the cause of the tiredness, since boredom in the group, lack of sleep, and physical illness are all possible reasons, each one requiring a different trainer response.

Active Resistance

Participation, but Not as Instructed. Trainees displaying this type of group management problem are "off target." They may be trying to role play, serve as coactor, give accurate feedback, or engage in other tasks required in skillstreaming, but their own personal agendas or mis-perceptions interfere, and they wander off course to irrelevant topics.

Passive–Aggressive Isolation. Passive–aggressive isolation is not just apathy, in which trainees are simply not interested in participating. Nor is it participation but not as instructed, in which trainees actively go off task and raise personal agendas. Passive–aggressive isolation is the purposeful, intentional withholding of appropriate participation, an active shutting down of involvement. It can be thought of as a figura-tive crossing of one's arms in order to display deliberate nonpartici-pation.

Negativism. When displaying negativism, trainees signal more overtly, by word and deed, their wish to avoid participation in the skill-streaming group. They may openly refuse to role play, provide feed-back, or complete homework assignments. Or, they may not come to sessions, come late to sessions, or walk out in the middle of sessions.

Disruptiveness. Disruptiveness encompasses active resistance be-haviors more extreme than negativism, such as openly and perhaps energetically ridiculing the trainers, other trainees, or aspects of the skillstreaming process. Or, disruptiveness may be shown by gestures, movements, noises, or other distracting nonverbal behaviors charac-teristically symbolizing overt criticism and hostility.

Hyperactivity

Digression. Digression is related to what we've called participation, but not as instructed. It is however a more repetitive, more determined, and more strongly motivated moving away from the purposes and procedures of skillstreaming. Here, the trainees are feeling some emo-tion strongly, such as anger or anxiety or despair, and are determined to express it. Or the skill portrayed by the trainers or other trainees may set off associations with important recent experiences, which the trainees feel the need to present and discuss. Digression is also often characterized by jumping out of role in the role play. Rather than merely wandering off track, in digression the trainees *drive* the train off its in-tended course.

Monopolizing. Monopolizing involves subtle and not-so-subtle ef-forts by trainees to get more than a fair share of time during a skill-streaming session. Long monologues, requests by the trainees to unnecessarily role play again, elaborate feedback, and attention-seeking efforts to remain on stage are examples of such monopolizing behavior.

Interruption. Similar to monopolizing, but more intrusive and in-sistent, interruption is literally breaking into the ongoing flow of a modeling display, role play, or feedback period with comments, questions, suggestions, observations, or other statements. Interruptions may be overly assertive or angry on the one hand, or may take a more pseudobenevolent guise of being offered by a "trainer's helper." In either event, such interruptions more often than not retard the group's progress toward its goals.

Excessive Restlessness. This is a more extreme, more physical form of hyperactivity. The trainees may fidget while sitting, rock their chairs, get up and pace, smoke a great deal, drink soft drinks one after the other, or display other nonverbal, verbal, gestural, or postural signs of restlessness. Such behavior will typically be accompanied by digressing, monopolizing, or interrupting behavior.

Cognitive Inadequacies and Emotional Disturbance

Inability to Pay Attention. Closely related to excessive restlessness, the inability to pay attention is often the result of internal or external distractions, daydreaming, or other pressing agendas that command the trainees' attention. Inability to pay attention except for brief periods of time may also be due to one or more forms of cognitive impairment.

Inability to Understand. Cognitive deficits due to developmental disability, intellectual inadequacy, impoverishment of experience, disease processes, or other sources may result in some aspect of the skillstreaming process not being understood, or being misunderstood, by the trainees. Failure to understand can, of course, also result from errors in the clarity and complexity of statements presented by the trainers.

Inability to Remember. Material presented in the skillstreaming group may be both attended to and understood by the trainees, but not remembered. This may result not only in problems of skill transfer and maintenance, but also in group management problems when what is forgotten includes rules and procedures for trainee participation, homework assignments, and so forth.

Bizarre Behavior. This type of group management problem is rare, but when instances of it do occur it can be especially disruptive to group functioning. It may not only pull other trainees off task but may frighten them or make them highly anxious. The range of bizarre behaviors is broad, and includes talking to oneself or inanimate objects, offering incoherent statements to the group, becoming angry for no apparent reason, hearing and responding to imaginary voices, and exhibiting peculiar mannerisms.

Reducing Group Management Problems

Most skillstreaming sessions proceed rather smoothly, but the competent trainer is a prepared trainer. Preparation includes knowing what problems might occur, as well as which corrective steps to take when they do occur.

Simplification Methods

Reward Minimal Trainee Accomplishments. Problematic trainee behavior can sometimes be altered by a process similar to what has been called "shaping." For example, rather than responding positively to trainees only when they enact a complete and accurate role play, reward in the form of praise and approval may be offered for lesser, but still successful, accomplishments. Perhaps only one or two behavioral steps were role played correctly. Or, in the extreme example of rewarding minimal trainee accomplishment, praise may be offered for "trying" after a totally unsuccessful role play or even for merely paying attention to someone else's role play.

Shorten the Role Play. A more direct means for simplifying the trainees' task is to ask less of them. One way of doing so is to shorten the role play, usually by asking trainees to role play only some (or one) of the behavioral steps that constitute the skill being taught.

Have Trainer "Feed" Sentences to the Trainee. With trainees having a particularly difficult time participating appropriately in the skillstreaming group, especially for reasons of cognitive inadequacy, the trainer may elect to take on the role of coach or prompter. There are a variety of ways this may be accomplished, perhaps the most direct of which involves a trainer standing immediately behind the trainee and whispering the statements that constitute proper enactment of each behavioral step for the trainee to then say out loud.

Have Trainee Read a Prepared Script. We have never used this approach, but others report some success with it. In essence, it removes the burden of figuring out what to say from the trainees and makes it easier for them to get up in front of the group and act out the skill's behavioral steps. Clearly, as with all simplification methods, using a prepared script should be seen as a temporary device, used to move trainees in the direction of role playing with no such special assistance from the trainers.

Have Trainee Play Coactor Role First. Another way to ease trainees into the responsibility of being a main actor is to have them first play the role of the coactor. This accustoms them more gradually to getting up before the group and speaking because the spotlight is mostly on someone else. As with the use of a prepared script, this method should be used only temporarily. Before moving on to the next skill, all trainees must always take on the role of the main actor with the particular skill.

Elicitation of Response Methods

Call for Volunteers. Particularly in the early stages of the life of a skillstreaming group, trainee participation may have to be actively elicited by the group's trainers. As trainees experience the group's procedures, find them personally relevant and valuable, and find support and acceptance from the trainers and from other group members, the need for such elicitation typically diminishes. The least directive form of such trainer activity is the straightforward calling for volunteers.

Introduce Topics for Discussion. Calling for volunteers, essentially an invitation to the group as a whole, may yield no response in a highly apathetic group. Under this circumstance, introducing topics for the group to discuss that appear relevant to the needs, concerns, aspirations, and particular skill deficiencies of the participating members will often be an effective course of action to pursue.

Call on a Specific Trainee. The largely nondirective elicitation methods already presented may be followed by a more active and directive trainer intervention if unsuccessful, that is, calling upon a particular trainee and requesting that trainee's participation. In doing so, it is often useful to select a trainee whose attentiveness, facial expression, eye contact, or other nonverbal signaling communicates potential involvement and interest.

Reinstruct Trainees by Means of Prompting and Coaching. The trainer may have to become still more active and directive and, in a manner similar to our earlier discussion of feeding role play lines to a trainee, prompt and coach the trainee to adequate participation. Such assistance may involve any aspect of the skillstreaming process — attending to the modeling display, following a skill's behavioral steps during the role playing, providing useful performance feedback after someone else's role play, completing the homework assignments in the proper manner, and so forth.

Threat Reduction Methods

Employ Additional Live Modeling by the Trainers. When the skillstreaming trainers engage in live modeling of the session's skill, they are doing more than just the main task of skill enactment. Such trainer behavior also makes it easier for trainees to similarly get up and risk less-than-perfect performances in an effort to learn the skill. For trainees who are particularly anxious, inhibited, or reluctant to role play, an additional portrayal or two of the same skill by the trainers may put them at ease. Such additional live modeling will also prove useful to those trainees having difficulty role playing because of cognitive inadequacies.

Postpone Trainee's Role Playing until Last. This recommendation is a straightforward extension of the tactic just presented. The threat of role playing may be reduced if a trainee is not required to role play until both the trainers' live modeling and the role playing by all other trainees are completed. It is crucial, though, that no trainee deficient in the session's skill be excused completely from role playing that skill. To do so would run counter to the central, skill-training purpose of skillstreaming.

Provide Reassurance to the Trainee. This method of dealing with group management problems involves the trainers' providing one or more trainees with brief, straightforward, simple, but very often highly effective, messages of encouragement and reassurance. "You can do it," "We'll help you as you go along," "Take it a step at a time" are but a few examples of such valuable reassurance.

Provide Empathic Encouragement to the Trainee. This is a method we have used often, with good results. In the case of trainee reluctance to role play, for example, the trainer may provide empathic encouragement by proceeding through the following steps:

Step 1: Offer the resistant trainee the opportunity to explain in greater detail his or her reluctance to role play and listen nondefensively.

Step 2: Clearly express your understanding of the resistant trainee's feelings.

Step 3: If appropriate, respond that the trainee's view is a viable alternative.

Step 4: Present your own view in greater detail, with both supporting reasons and probable outcomes.

Step 5: Express the appropriateness of delaying a resolution of the trainer–trainee difference.

Step 6: Urge the trainee to try to role play the given behavioral steps.

The identical procedure may be used effectively with a wide range of other trainee resistances.

Clarify Threatening Aspects of the Trainee's Task. Clarifying threatening aspects of tasks requires deeper explanations, repetition of earlier clarifications, and provision of further illustrations. In all instances, the task involved remains unchanged, but what is required of trainees to complete the task is clarified.

Restructure Threatening Aspects of the Trainee's Task. Unlike the method just discussed, in which the task remains unchanged and the trainers seek to clarify the trainee's understanding of it, in the present method the trainers may alter the trainee's task if it is seen as threatening. Behavioral steps may be altered, simplified, moved around, deleted, or added. Role plays may be shortened, lengthened, changed in content, merged with other skills, or otherwise changed. Aspects of performance feedback may be changed, too—the sequence of who delivers it, its generality versus specificity, its timing, its length, its focus. No aspect of skillstreaming should be considered unchangeable. All treatment, training, and teaching methods should be open to revision as needed in the judgment of their skilled and sensitive users. Most certainly, this also includes skillstreaming.

Termination of Response Methods

Urge Trainee to Remain on Task. Gently, but firmly, trainers may retrieve trainees who wander off the group's task by reminding, cajoling, admonishing, or simply clearly pointing out to trainees what they are doing incorrectly and what they ought to be doing instead.

Ignore Trainee Behavior. Certain inappropriate trainee behaviors can be terminated most effectively by simply ignoring them. This withdrawal of reinforcement, or extinction process, is best applied to those problem behaviors that the group can tolerate while still remaining on task during the extinction process. Behaviors such as pacing, whispering to oneself, and occasional interruptions are examples of behaviors best terminated by simply ignoring them. Behaviors that are more disruptive to the group's functioning, or may be dangerous, will have to be dealt with more directly.

Interrupt Ongoing Trainee Behavior. This method requires directive and assertive trainer behavior. We recommend interrupting ongoing trainee behavior primarily when other methods fail. Interrupting trainees' inappropriate, erroneous, or disruptive behavior should be carried out firmly, unequivocally, and with the clear message that the group has its tasks and they must be gotten on with. In its extreme form, interrupting trainee behavior may even require removing trainees from groups for a brief, or for an extended, period of time.

Trainee Motivation

Which skills shall be taught, and who will select them? This is as much a motivational as a tactical question, for to the degree the youngster can expect to learn skill competencies that he or she thinks are presently deficient, but can be very useful in real world relationships, his or her motivation is correspondingly enhanced. We have operationalized this perspective by means of a process we call "negotiating the curriculum." Skills trainer and trainee compare, contrast, examine, and select from their skills inventories in such a manner that trainer beliefs about what the trainee needs, and trainee beliefs about his or her own deficiencies and desired competencies are mutually reflected.

Where are the group sessions held? In addition to these intrinsic motivators, certain group parameters may be varied to act as extrinsic motivators for learning new skills. In most schools and institutions we try to use a special place, associated in the trainee's thinking with particular privileges or opportunities, (e.g., teacher's lounge, student center, recreational area), and yet not a place so removed in its characteristics from the typical application settings in which trainees function as to reduce the likelihood of skill transfer.

When will the group meet? If it is not too great an academic sacrifice, we attempt to schedule school-based skills training sessions when the youngsters will have to miss an activity he or she does not especially enjoy—including certain academic subjects—rather than free play, lunch, gym, or the like.

Who will lead the group? Particularly for the beginning sessions of our initial groups, we try to use as trainers those teachers, cottage parents, members of the institutional staff, or others who seem to be most stimulating, most tuned to the needs and behaviors of aggressive adolescents (but not the most overtly empathic), and in general most able to capture and hold the attention of participating youngsters. This strategy often has beneficial motivational consequences for both the initial groups of trainees and, through the school's or institution's grapevine, subsequent groups of trainees.

Which skill shall be taught first? The first skill taught should be one that is likely to yield immediate, real world reward for the trainee. It must work; it must pay off. While some trainers prefer to begin with the simpler conversational skills as a sort of warm-up or break-in, our preference is to try to respond to both simplicity and reward potential.

This consideration of trainee motivation completes our presentation of the procedures that constitute skillstreaming. We turn now to the further psychological skills training intervention groupings into which skillstreaming has evolved. First we will examine aggression replacement training, and then the Prepare Curriculum.

AGGRESSION REPLACEMENT TRAINING

As noted earlier, the frequent failure of transfer or maintenance of training gains is a common outcome not only across skills training approaches but in interventions of all types (Goldstein & Kanfer, 1979; Karoly & Steffan, 1980; Keeley, Chemberg, & Carbonell, 1976). This common failure of such gains to generalize across settings or time formed the primary motivation for our effort to expand our intervention beyond skillstreaming alone to an expanded program of aggression replacement training. Many efforts designed to enhance transfer and maintenance have appropriately turned outward—to parents, employers, teachers, siblings or other benign and gain-reinforcing persons available in the trainees' real world environments. One is rarely so fortunate with the type of trainee upon whom most of our work has focused: chronically aggressive youth. Far too often parents are indifferent or unavailable; peers are the original tutors of antisocial, not prosocial, behavior; employers are nonexistent or too busy; and teachers have written the youngsters off years ago. To be sure, when and if the assistance of such persons can be mobilized, one should energetically do so. Much more often, however, one is left with but a single transfer and maintenance enhancement option; that is, working directly with the youngster. If skillstreaming alone fails to provide reliable transfer and maintenance outcomes, we reasoned, then our intervention must be broadened and its coverage and potency increased, in a fuller effort to arm the youngster with whatever is needed to learn to behave in constructive, nonaggressive, and still-satisfying ways in the classroom and community. With this as our guiding philosophy, we constructed and evaluated *aggression replacement training*, a three-component training intervention.

1. *Skillstreaming.* As noted above, skillstreaming is a systematic, psychoeducational intervention demonstrated across a great many investigations for the purpose of reliably teaching a 50-skill curriculum of prosocial behaviors. In addition to other target behaviors, it teaches youngsters behaviors they may use instead of aggression in response to provocations they may experience.

2. *Anger control training.* Developed by Feindler and her research group (Feindler, Marriott, & Iwata, 1984), and based in part on the sem-

inal anger control and stress inoculation research, of Novaco (1975) and Meichenbaum (1977), anger control training — in contrast to skillstreaming's goal of prosocial behavior facilitation — teaches the self-regulation and inhibition of anger, aggression, and, more generally, antisocial behavior. By breaking behavior into its constituent parts — for example, identify the physiological cues of anger and its external and internal triggers, initiating self-statement disputation training, refocusing anticipation or consequences, and so forth — chronically angry and aggressive youth are taught to respond to provocation (others and their own) less impulsively, more reflectively, and with less likelihood of acting-out behavior. In short, anger control training teaches youngsters what not to do in anger-instigating situations.

3. *Moral education*. Armed with both the ability to respond to the real world prosocially, and the skills necessary to stifle impulsive anger and aggression, will the chronically acting-out youngster in fact choose to do so? To enhance that likelihood, we believe that moral values must come into play.

In a long and pioneering series of investigations, Kohlberg (1969, 1973) has demonstrated that exposing youngsters to a series of moral dilemmas, in the context of a discussion-group that includes youngsters reasoning at differing levels of moral thinking, arouses an experience of cognitive conflict whose resolution will frequently advance a youngster's moral reasoning to that of the higher level peers in the group. While this is a reliable finding, as with other single interventions, efforts to use it by itself have yielded only mixed success (Arbuthnot & Gordon, 1983; Zimmerman, 1983) — perhaps because such youngsters did not have in their behavior repertoires either the skill behaviors needed for acting prosocially or for successfully inhibiting the antisocial. We thus reasoned that Kohlbergian moral education has marked potential for providing constructive motivation toward prosocialness and away from antisocialness in youngsters armed with the benefits of both skillstreaming and anger control training.

Our four evaluations of the efficacy of aggression replacement training employed with chronically aggressive, delinquent youth each yielded positive findings (Goldstein & Glick, 1987; Goldstein, Glick, Irwin, Pask, & Rubama, 1989). To build further upon such outcomes, we have moved recently beyond aggression replacement training to a new, more comprehensive expression of this psychological skills training intervention philosophy, which we call the Prepare Curriculum (Goldstein, 1989).

THE PREPARE CURRICULUM

The first three courses of this 10-course intervention are the three components that constitute aggression replacement training, described
above. Thus, Course 1 is skillstreaming. Course 2 is anger control training, and Course 3 is moral education. A description of the remaining
seven courses follows.

Course 4. Problem-Solving Training

Aggressive adolescents and younger children are frequently deficient
not only in using such prosocial competencies as the array of interpersonal skills and anger control techniques taught in Courses 1 and 2,
but they may also be deficient in other skills essential to prosocial behavior. They may, as Ladd and Mize (1983) point out, be deficient in
such problem-solving competencies as "(a) knowledge of appropriate
goals for social interaction, (b) knowledge of appropriate *strategies* for
reaching a social goal, and (c) knowledge of the *contexts* in which specific
strategies may be appropriately applied" (p. 130).

An analogous conclusion flows from the research program on interpersonal problem solving conducted by Spivack, Platt and Shure
(1976). In early and middle childhood, as well as in adolescence, chronically aggressive youngsters were less able than more typical youngsters
to function effectively in most problem-solving subskills, such as identifying alternatives, considering consequences, determining causality,
means–ends thinking, and perspective taking.

Several programs have been developed in an effort to remedy such
problem-solving deficiencies with the types of youngsters of concern
here (DeLange, Lanham, & Barton, 1981; Giebink, Stover, & Fahl, 1968;
Sarason & Sarason, 1981). Such programs represent a fine beginning,
but problem-solving deficiencies in such youth are substantial (Chandler, 1973; Selman, 1980; Spivack et al., 1976), and require substantial,
longer-term, more comprehensive interventions. The Prepare Curriculum problem-solving training course, outlined in Table 3.1, seeks to
provide just such an intervention. It is a longer-term (than existing programs) sequence of such graduated problem-solving skills as reflection,
problem identification, information gathering, identification of alternatives, consideration of consequences and decision making. Our initial evaluation of this sequence with an aggressive adolescent population
has yielded significant gains in the problem-solving skills thus defined,
substantially encouraging further development of this course (Grant,
1987). These results provide an initial basis for our earlier assertion that

TABLE 3.1. Prepare Curriculum Course 4: Problem-Solving Training

Session 1	Introduction
Session 2	Stop and think
Session 3	Problem identification
Session 4	Gathering information (own perspective)
Session 5	Gathering information (other's perspective)
Session 6	Identifying alternatives
Session 7	Evaluating consequences
Session 8	Review and practice

individuals can be provided systematic training in problem solving skills both for purposes of building general competence in meeting life's challenges, and as a specific means of supplying one more reliable, prosocial alternative to aggression. (Goldstein, 1988, p. 43)

Course 5. Empathy Training

We especially wanted to include a course designed to enhance the participating youth's level of empathy because the expression of empathic understanding can simultaneously serve as an inhibitor of negative interactions and facilitator of positive ones. Evidence shows that

> responding to another individual in an empathic manner and assuming temporarily their perspective decreases or inhibits one's potential for acting aggressively toward the other (Feshbach, 1982; Feshbach & Feshbach, 1969). Stated otherwise, empathy and aggression are incompatible interpersonal responses, hence to be more skilled in the former serves as an aid to diminishing the latter. (Goldstein & Michaels, 1985, p. 309)

The notion of empathy as a facilitator of positive interpersonal relations stands on an even broader base of research evidence. Our recent review of the hundreds of investigations of the interpersonal consequences of empathic responding reveal such responding to be a consistently potent promotor of interpersonal attraction, dyadic openness, conflict resolution, and individual growth (Goldstein & Michaels, 1985). It is a most potent facilitator indeed.

This same review led us to define empathy as a multistage process of perceiving emotional cues, the affective reverberation of those cues, and their cognitive labeling and communication. Correspondingly, we developed the Prepare Curriculum multistage training program by which these four components could be taught. This program is presented in outline form in Table 3.2, and in detail in the text, the Prepare Curriculum (Goldstein, 1988).

Course 6. Situational Perception Training

Once armed with the interpersonal skills necessary to respond prosocially to others (Courses 1, 2, and 3), the problem-solving strategies underlying skill selection and usage (Course 4), and a fuller, empathic sense of the other person's perspective (Course 5), the chronically aggressive youngster may still fail to behave prosocially because he or she misreads the context in which behavior is to occur. A major thrust in psychology in the past 15 years has been this emphasis on *the situation or setting, as perceived by the individual,* and its importance in determining overt behavior. Morrison and Bellack (1981) comment, for example,

> adequate social performance not only requires a repertoire of response skills, but knowledge about when and how these responses should be applied. Application of this knowledge, in turn, depends upon the ability to accurately "read" the social environment: determine the particular norms and conventions operating at the moment, and to understand the messages being sent . . . and intentions guiding the behavior of the interpersonal partner. (p. 70)

Dil (1972), Emery (1975), and Rothenberg (1970) have shown that emotionally disturbed youngsters, as well as those who are socially maladjusted in other ways are characteristically deficient in such social perceptiveness. Furnham and Argyle (1981) observe,

> It has been found that people who are socially inadequate are unable to read everyday situations and respond appropriately. They are unable to perform or interpret nonverbal signals, unaware of the rules of social behavior, mystified by ritualized routines and conventions of self-presentation and self-disclosure, and are hence like foreigners in their own land. (p. 37)

Argyle, Furnham, and Graham (1981) and Backman (1979) have stressed this same social–perceptual deficit in their work with aggressive individuals. Dodge, Price, Bachorowski, and Newman (1990) have done similarly, especially with reference to aggressive adolescents. In their study of the "cycle of violence" they found that

> harmed children are likely to develop biased and deficient patterns of processing social information, including a failure to attend to relevant

TABLE 3.2. Empathy Training: A Components Approach

I. Readiness training
   1. Acquisition of empathy preparatory skills (Frank, 1977)
      a. Imagination skills: to increase accurate identification of implied meanings
      b. Behavioral observation skills: to increase accurate prediction of others' overt behavior
      c. Flexibility skills: to increase differentiation ability in shifting from (a) to (b)
   2. Elimination of empathy skill acquisition inhibitors
      a. Programmed self-instruction to understand one's perceptual biases (Bullmer, 1972)
      b. Interpersonal process recall: to reduce affect-associated anxiety (Pereira, 1978).

II. Perceptual training
   1. Programmed self-instruction (Bullmer, 1972): to increase interpersonal perceptual accuracy and objectivity
   2. Observational sensitivity training (Smith, 1973): to increase competence in recording sensory impressions, and discriminate them from inferential, interpretive impressions

III. Affective reverberation training
   1. Mediation (Goleman, 1977; Lesh, 1970)
   2. Structural integration or Rolfing (Keen, 1970; Rolf, 1977)
   3. Reichian therapy (Lowen, 1967; Reich, 1933/1949)
   4. Bioenergetics (Lowen & Lowen, 1977)
   5. Alexander technique (Alexander, 1969)
   6. Feldenkrais' Awareness Through Movement (Feldenkrais, 1970, 1972)
   7. Dance therapy (Bernstein, 1975; Pesso, 1969)
   8. Sensory awareness training (Brooks, 1974; Gunther, 1968)
   9. Focusing (Gendlin, 1981, 1984)
   10. Laban–Bartenieff method (Bartenieff & Lewis, 1980)

IV. Cognitive analysis training
   1. Discrimination training (Carkhuff, 1969) in utilizing perceptual (II) and reverberatory (III) information
   2. Exposure (to e.g., facial expressions) plus guided practice and feedback on affective labeling accuracy (Allport, 1924; Davitz, 1964)

V. Communication training
   1. Didactic–experiential training (Carkhuff, 1969)
   2. Interpersonal living laboratory (Egan, 1976)
   3. Relationship enhancement (Guerney, 1977)
   4. Microtraining: Enriching intimacy program (Ivey & Authier, 1971)
   5. Structured learning training (Goldstein, 1981)

VI. Transfer and maintenance training
   1. Provision of general principles (Duncan, 1953; Judd, 1902)
   2. Maximizing identical elements (Osgood, 1953; Thorndike & Woodworth, 1901)
   3. Maximizing response availability (Mandler, 1954; Underwood & Schultz, 1960)
   4. Maximizing stimulus variability (Callantine & Warren, 1955; Shore & Sechrest, 1961)
   5. Programmed, real-world reinforcement (Galassi & Galassi, 1984)

Note. From Goldstein (1988). Copyright 1988 Arnold P. Goldstein. Reprinted by permission.

cues, a bias to attribute hostile intention to others, and a lack of competent behavioral strategies to solve interpersonal problems. These patterns,
in turn, were found to predict the development of aggressive behavior.
(p. 390)

We believe that the ability to accurately read social situations can be
taught. To accomplish this goal, this course's contents are responsive
to the valuable leads provided in this context by Brown and Fraser
(1979) who propose three salient dimensions of accurate social perceptiveness: (1) the *setting* of the interaction and its associated rules and
norms, (2) the *purpose* of the interaction and its goals, tasks, and topics,
and (3) the *relationship* of the participants, their roles, responsibilities,
expectations, and group memberships. Concretely, situational perception training requires that trainees be confronted with an array of relevant, difficult situational descriptions and, employing a problem-solving
group process (i.e., Prepare Curriculum Course 4), (1) identify situational characteristics (e.g., rules, roles, goals) useful in reducing situational difficulty, (2) generate alternative means for accomplishing such
reduction of conflict or difficulty, (3) select from among these means,
and (4) evaluate likely alternative outcomes.

Course 7. Stress Management

We have oriented each of the preceding course descriptions toward
either directly enhancing prosocial competency (e.g., skillstreaming,
moral reasoning, social perceptiveness), or reducing qualities that inhibit previously learned or newly acquired prosocial competency (e.g.,
anger control training). The course we will now describe is of this latter type. It has been demonstrated by Arkowitz, Lichtenstein, McGovern,
and Hines (1975) and Curran (1977) that individuals may possess an
array of prosocial skills in their repertoires, but not employ them in
particularly challenging or difficult situations because of anxiety. A
youth may have learned well the skillstreaming skill Responding to
Failure, but embarrassment at getting a failing grade in front of the
teacher or missing a foul shot in front of friends may engender a level
of anxiety that inhibits proper use of this skill. A young woman may
possess the problem-solving competency to plan well for a job interview, but perform poorly in the interview itself as anxiety takes over.
Such anxiety/inhibition as a source of prosocially incompetent and un-
satisfying behavior may be especially prevalent in the high peer-
conscious adolescent years.

   This stress-induced anxiety may be substantially reduced by fol-

TABLE 3.3. Prepare Curriculum Course 7:
Stress Management Training

1. Progressive relaxation training
2. Yogaform stretching
3. Breathing exercises
4. Physical exercises
5. Somatic focusing
6. Thematic imagery
7. Meditation

lowing the procedures that form the contents of the Prepare Curriculum stress management course. As outlined in Table 3.3, participating youngsters are taught systematic deep muscular relaxation. (Benson, 1975; Jacobson, 1964), meditation techniques (Assagioli, 1973; Naranjo & Ornstein, 1971), environmental restructuring (Anderson, 1978), exercise (Walker, 1975), and related means for the management, control, and reduction of stress.

Course 8. Cooperation Training

Chronically aggressive youths have been shown to display a personality trait pattern quite often high in egocentricity and competitiveness, and low in concern for others and cooperativeness (Pepitone, 1985; Slavin et al., 1985). We offer a course in cooperation training not only because enhanced cooperation among individuals is a valuable social goal, but also because of the several valuable concomitants and consequences of enhanced cooperation. An extended review of research on one major set of approaches to cooperation training, namely cooperative learning, reveals outcomes of enhanced self-esteem, group cohesiveness, altruism and cooperation itself, as well as reduced egocentricity. As long ago as 1929, Maller commented,

> The frequent staging of contests, the constant emphasis upon the making and breaking of record, and the glorification of the heroic individual achievement . . . in our present educational system lead toward the acquisition of competitiveness. The child is trained to look at members of his group as constant competitors and urged to put forth a maximum effort to excel them. The lack of practice in group activities and community projects in which the child works with his fellows for a common goal precludes the formation of habits of cooperativeness. . . . (p. 163)

It was many years before the educational establishment responded concretely to this Deweyian-like challenge, but when it did it created a wide series of innovative, cooperation-enhancing methodologies,
each of which deserves long and careful application and scrutiny both
in general educational contexts and, as in our case, with particularly
noncooperative youth. We refer to the cooperative learning methods
listed in Table 3.4. Using shared materials, interdependent tasks, group
rewards, and similar features, these methods (applied to any content
area—mathematics, social studies, etc.) have consistently yielded the
several interpersonal, cooperation-enhancing, group and individual
benefits noted above.

In developing our course, we sorted through existing methods, adding touches of our own, and prescriptively tailored a cooperative learning course sequence of special value for chronically aggressive youth.
We made use not only of the many valuable features of the cooperative learning approaches noted above but, in addition, responded to
the physical action orientation typical of such youths by relying heavi-

---

TABLE 3.4. Prepare Curriculum Course 8: Cooperation Training

A. Cooperative learning methods
   1. Student teams—achievement divisions (Slavin, 1980)
   2. Teams—games—tournaments (Slavin, 1980)
   3. Team assisted individualization (Slavin, Leavey, & Medden, 1982)
   4. Jigsaw I (Aronson, Blaney, Stephan, Sikes, & Snapp, 1978)
   5. Jigsaw II (Slavin, 1980)
   6. Learning togther (Johnson & Johnson, 1975)
   7. Group investigation (Sharan, Raviv, & Russell, 1982)
   8. Co-op co-op (Kagan, 1985)

B. Cooperative gaming
   1. Ages 3–7:
      a. Jack-in-the-box name game
      b. Cooperative hide-and-seek
      c. Partner gymnastics
      d. Frozen bean bags
   2. Ages 8–12:
      a. New basketball
      b. Three-sided soccer
      c. Tug of peace
      d. All on one side
   3. Adolescent:
      a. Strike-outless baseball
      b. Mutual storytelling
      c. Octopus massage
      d. Brussels sprouts

Note. From Goldstein (1988). Copyright 1988 Arnold P. Goldstein. Reprinted by permission.

ly on cooperative sports and games. Such athletic activity, while not popular in the United States, does exist elsewhere in both action and written document (Orlick, 1978a, 1978b, 1982; Fluegelman, 1981). Collective-score basketball, no hitting football, cross-team rotational hockey, collective-fastest-time track meets and other sports restructured to be what cooperative gaming creators term "all touch" "all play" "all positions" "all shoot," may seem strange to the typical American youth, weaned on highly competitive, individualistic sports. But we think this will be a valuable additional approach to be use with aggressive youth as we work toward the goal of cooperation enhancement. In Table 3.4 we have listed a few of the several dozen such activities which are part of this Prepare Curriculum course (Goldstein, 1988).

Course 9. Recruiting Supportive Models

Aggressive youths are typically exposed to highly aggressive models; in parents, siblings, and peers are often chronically aggressive individuals themselves (Knight & West, 1975; Loeber & Dishion, 1983; Osborn & West, 1979; Robins, West, & Herjanic, 1975). At the samem time, there tend to be relatively few, countervailing prosocial models available to be observed and imitated. When they are, however, such prosocial models can apparently make a tremendous difference in the daily lives and development of such youth. Accordingly, we may turn to such community-provided examples of prosocial modeling as Big Brothers, the Police Athletic League, or Boy Scouts, and the like. And we not only examine the laboratory research consistently showing that rewarded prosocial behaviors (e.g., sharing, altruism, cooperation) are quite often imitated (Bryan & Test, 1967; Evers & Schwarz, 1973; Canale, 1977), but we look at more direct evidence as well. For example, Werner and Smith (1982), in their impressive longitudinal study of aggressive and nonaggressive youth, *Vulnerable but Invincible,* clearly demonstrated that many youngsters growing up in a community characterized by high crime, high unemployment, high school drop-out rates, and high numbers of aggressive models, were indeed able to develop into effective, satisfied, prosocially oriented individuals if they had had sustained exposure to at least one significant prosocial model, be it parent, relative, or peer. Similar results have been reported by Ellis and Lane (1978), Hawkins and Fraser (1983), Kauffman, Gruenbaum, Cohler, and Gamer (1979), and Pines (1979).

Since such models are often scarce in the real world environments of the youths the Prepare Curriculum is intended to serve, efforts must be put forth to help these young people identify, encourage, attract, elicit, and at times perhaps even create attachments to others who not only function prosocially themselves, but who can also serve as sustained sources of support for their own prosocially oriented efforts.

Our course content for teaching such skills relies in large part on both the teaching procedures and certain of the interpersonal skills that constitute our skillstreaming skills training curriculum for adolescents (Goldstein et al., 1980) and younger children (McGinnis & Goldstein, 1984; e.g., Prepare Curriculum Course 1).

Course 10. Understanding and Using Group Processes

Adolescent and preadolescent acute responsiveness to peer influences is a truism frequently expressed in both lay and professional literature on child development. It is a conclusion resting on a solid research foundation (Baumrind, 1975; Field, 1981; Guralnick, 1981; Manaster, 1977; Moriarty & Toussieng, 1976; Rosenberg, 1975). As a curriculum designed to enhance prosocial competencies, it is especially important that the Prepare Curriculum include a segment giving special emphasis to group—especially peer group—processes. Its title includes both "understanding" and "using" because both are clearly its goals. Participating youth will be helped to understand such group forces and phenomena as peer pressure, clique formation and dissolution, leaders and leadership, cohesiveness, imitation, reciprocity, in-group versus out-group relations, developmental phases, competition, within-group communication and its failure, and similar processes.

For such understanding to have real world value for participating youth (the "using" component of our course title), this course's instructional format consists almost exclusively of group activities in which participants can learn *experientially* the means for effectively resisting group pressure when one elects to do so, for seeking and enacting a group leadership role, for helping build and enjoy the fruits of group cohesiveness, and so forth. Examples drawn from the several dozen specific Prepare Curriculum activities which constitute this course are listed in Table 3.5.

SUMMARY

We have evaluated and described three sequentially more comprehensive psychological skills training interventions. Their successful employment with chronically aggressive youths is well established. Their continued use and systematic evaluation is strongly to be encouraged.

TABLE 3.5. The Prepare Curriculum
Course 10: Group Dynamics

A. Forming
   1. Who am I? A getting acquainted activity
   2. Group conversation: discussion starters
   3. Group development: a graphic analysis
   4. Verbal activities within groups

B. Storming
   1. Conflict resolution: a collection of tasks
   2. Discrimination: simulation activities
   3. Rumor clinic
   4. Nonverbal communication

C. Norming
   1. Group self-evaluations
   2. Group-on-group: a feedback experience
   3. Styles of leadership
   4. Dyadic encounter

D. Performing
   1. Top problems: a consensus-seeking task
   2. Line up and power inversion
   3. Stretching: identifying and taking risks
   4. Cash register: group decision making

E. Adjourning

NOTE

1. Also see Goldstein, Sprafkin, Gershaw, and Klein (1980) for skillstreaming procedures and materials for adolescents, McGinnis and Goldstein (1984) for elementary age children, and McGinnis and Goldstein (1990) for preschool children.

C H A P T E R   4

✛

Behavior Modification Techniques

In sum, the results of a decade or so of research have
documented the effectiveness of the behavior modification
approach in a wide variety of settings with very diverse
child populations. . . . The behavior of children in classroom
settings has been repeatedly altered by a variety of different
procedures used by a number of investigators. In contrast to
a host of other approaches applied to educational problems,
most behavioral principles . . . were first documented in
laboratory settings, and thus there is evidence from both
basic and applied research of the efficacy of such principles.
— K. D. O'Leary and S. G. O'Leary (1980, p. 17)

Though the bulk of this chapter consists of an examination of behavior
modification techniques of demonstrated effectiveness with aggressive
youngsters, their sound empirical bases are an overriding consideration for both understanding and developing these techniques, and for
making decisions about their adoption and implementation. The technology of behavior modification indeed rests upon a firm experimental foundation.

There are important reasons to include a chapter on behavior
modification other than the repeated demonstration that it works. Behavior modification techniques are relatively easy to learn and use; may
be teacher-, peer-, parent-, and/or self-administered; are generally cost
effective; yield typically unambiguous behavior-change results; have a
long history of successful application with aggressive youngsters; and,
for these reasons, can make more time available for teachers to do what
most teachers do best . . . teach!

That is the good news. Many see a darker, much less positive side to the behavior modification coin. Some of its techniques are viewed as bribery, and as likely to increase disruptive behaviors in class as non-disruptive youngsters see their more aggressive peers receive rewards for reducing their levels of disruptiveness. All behavior modification techniques, its critics hold further, are unfair, highly manipulative, mechanistic, overly simplistic, demanding of extra teacher effort, and generally promote a view of people as objects to be acted upon. We address these ethical and philosophical reservations and objections later in this chapter.

DEFINITIONS

Behavior modification is a set of techniques, derived from formal learning theory, systematically applied in an effort to change observable behavior, and rigorously evaluated by experimental research. Almost all of its constituent techniques derive from the premise developed by Skinner and his followers (Ferster & Skinner, 1957; Skinner, 1938, 1953) that behavior is largely determined by its consequences. In an operational sense, this premise has found expression in techniques that by one means or another contingently present or withdraw rewards or punishments (e.g., environmental consequences) in order to alter the behavior that precedes these consequences. This contingent quality has led to the use of the term *contingency management* to describe most of the activities in which the behavior modifier engages. Specifically, if one's goal is to *increase* the likelihood that a given (e.g., prosocial) behavior will occur, one follows instances of its occurrence with positive consequences, that is, by means of some technique for presenting a reward or removing an aversive event. If one's goal is to *decrease* the likelihood that a given (e.g., antisocial) behavior will occur, one follows instances of its occurrence with negative consequences, that is, by means of some technique for presenting an aversive event or removing a rewarding event. To decrease the disruptiveness, aggression, or acting-out behavior of a given youngster, and simultaneously increase the chances that he or she will behave in a constructive, attending, prosocial manner, the skilled behavior modifier will often use a combination of aversive or reward-withdrawing (for aggression) and aversiveness-reducing or reward-providing (for constructive behavior) techniques. A few formal definitions will clarify the substance of the contingency management process.

A *reinforcer* is an event that increases the subsequent frequency of any behavior it follows. When the presentation of an event following a behavior increases its frequency, the event is referred to as a *positive reinforcer*. Praise, special privileges, tokens or points exchangeable for toys or snacks are a few examples of positive reinforcers. When the removal of an event following a behavior increases the subsequent frequency of the behavior, the event is referred to as a *negative reinforcer*. When a youngster ceases to behave in a disruptive manner after the teacher yells at him or her to do so, we may say that the teacher was negatively reinforced, and thus the future likelihood of teacher yelling is increased. When the presentation of an event following a behavior decreases its subsequent frequency, the event is referred to as a *punisher*. In the preceding example, the teacher's yelling, which was negatively reinforced by the student's decrease in disruptive behavior, functions as a punishment to the student to the extent that it decreases the likelihood of subsequent student disruptiveness.

A second way of decreasing the probability of a given behavior is by removing positive reinforcers each time the behavior occurs. Ignoring the behavior or removing the reinforcer of attention (i.e., extinction), physically removing the person from important sources of reinforcement (i.e., time-out), and removing the reinforcers from the person (i.e., response cost) are three means of contingently managing behavior by removing positive reinforcers.

All of these four procedures are means for either presenting or removing aversive stimuli, but presenting or removing positive reinforcement is by far the more common use of contingency management in schools.

NONCLASSROOM APPLICATIONS

Though many of the ideas relevant to the contingency management approach to human behavior had existed for a number of years (Mower & Mower, 1938; Skinner, 1938; Watson & Rayner, 1920), it was not until the 1950s that they were implemented in hospitals, clinics, schools, and other institutions for disturbed or disturbing youngsters. Skinner's (1953) book *Science and Human Behavior* was a significant stimulus to this development, as were a large number of investigations conducted during the 1950s and 1960s. All of these demonstrated the behavior-change effectiveness of contingency management. Much of this research sought to alter the highly aggressive or otherwise severely deviant behavior of institutionalized emotionally disturbed, autistic, or developmentally disabled children and adolescents, and did so with considerable success (Ayllon & Michael, 1959; Ferster & DeMyer, 1962; Lovaas, Schaeffer, & Simmons, 1965; Wolf, Risley, & Mees, 1964). In outpatient clinic and laboratory settings, successful use of contingency management was reported with such diverse behaviors as delinquency rates (Patterson, Ray, & Shaw, 1968; Schwitzgebel, 1964), social withdrawal (Allen, Hart, Buell, Harris, & Wolf, 1964; Lovaas, Koegel, Simmons, & Long, 1973), fearfulness (Lazarus & Rachman, 1967; Patterson, 1965), hyperactivity (Allen, Kenke, Harris, Baer, & Reynolds, 1967; Hall, Lund, & Jackson, 1968), depression (Wahler & Pollio, 1968), anorexia (Bachrach, Erwin, & Mohr, 1965; Leitenberg, Agras, & Thomson, 1968), mutism (Sherman, 1965; Straughan, 1968), and dozens of other deviant behaviors involving hundreds of youngsters.

The success of this orientation to behavior change has increased further in the 1970s and 1980s, finding still wider application across many behaviors and settings. It is not surprising, given the breadth and depth of this successful demonstration of behavior-change effectiveness, that numerous studies evaluating the classroom application of contingency management were also forthcoming.

CLASSROOM USE:
CONTINGENCY MANAGEMENT PROCEDURES

Classroom use of contingency management begins with (1) selecting behavioral goals; (2) informing the class of the behavioral rules they are to follow in order to reach such goals; (3) observing and recording current (base rate) classroom behavior; and then (4) applying one or a combination of behavior-change procedures (the presentation or removal of either positive reinforcement or aversive stimuli) in order to alter undesirable current behaviors. In the rest of this chapter we examine each step in the process in detail.

SELECTING BEHAVIORAL GOALS

What should the behavioral climate of the classroom be? Which student behaviors are best defined by the teacher as truly disruptive and as impediments to learning, and which tolerated or even welcomed as normative, or possibly even as facilitative of the learning process? Behavior-change goal selection should concern itself with reducing those aggressive, disruptive, acting-out behaviors that interfere with the learning process, but it must also be acutely responsive to normal stages of student development, examined to the extent possible in collaboration with the students themselves. In addition, behavior modification should be appropriately responsive to both teacher needs and the influence of overall school policy on decisions about classroom decorum. Each reader must make his or her own decisions in this regard, but our position regarding behavioral goal setting is that it is better to err slightly on the side of permissiveness and underregulation than risk an overly rigid classroom climate that is likely to inhibit both aggression and learning. Sarason, Glaser, and Fargo (1972) reflect this sentiment well:

> Disruptive children can be managed, but if behavior modification is used to make children conform to a rigid idea of goodness or to squelch creativity or to force sterile compliance, the cost of an orderly classroom may be too high. Behavior modification is not intended to serve as a new type of tranquilizer. It is intended to serve as a means of facilitating efforts to bring about meaningful learning. (p. 13)

In addition to the influences of students, school policy, and the community (see Chapters 7 and 8) on the teacher's decisions about behavioral goals for the classroom, such goal selection can meaningfully follow from the teacher's answers to such questions as:

1. What kind of student behavior interferes with the learning of the rest of the class, and what is perhaps annoying to you but essentially harmless to the learner and his or her peers?
2. How much classroom freedom can be permitted without interfering with the rights of other students? On the other side of this coin, what are your responsibilities and the responsibilities of the students?
3. Should silence be maintained while children are working, or should reasonable communication among students be permitted, such as is encouraged in the "open classroom"?
4. Are your classroom regulations really for the benefit of the students . . . or primarily for your own comfort and convenience?
5. Are you thinking about how the disruptive child can be helped to learn better, not just how the disruptive behavior can be decreased?
6. Have you been able to maintain an attitude of openness to new ideas and approaches that can benefit children even though they do not coincide with your personal biases?
7. Have you considered the attitudes and standards of the child and his or her family in setting standards for the child? Are your standards in conflict with theirs?
8. Have you discussed your goals for the class with the class?
9. Have you discussed your goals for the child with the child and his or her parents? (Sarason et al., 1972, p. 23)

These questions are often hard questions to answer, but they reflect the fact that the teacher is primary among several determiners of class-room behavior. Given this, we urge that goals be selected in a careful, thoughtful, ethical manner in which conduciveness to learning is the central criterion.

COMMUNICATING BEHAVIORAL RULES

Having decided the behavioral directions in which a class is to head, particularly with regard to reducing aggressive and disruptive behaviors and increasing positive behaviors, the teacher's next task is to communicate clearly to the students the rules and procedures they are to follow in order to attain these goals. A number of effective "rules for use of rules" have emerged in the contingency management literature (Greenwood, Hops, Delquadri, & Guild, 1974; Sarason et al., 1972; Walker, 1979), and include:

1. *Define and communicate rules for student behavior in clear, specific, behavioral terms.* As Walker (1979) notes, it is better (more concrete and behavioral) to say "Raise your hand before asking a question" than "Be considerate of others." Similarly, "Listen carefully to teacher instructions" or "Pay attention to the assignment and complete your work" are more likely to serve as rules that actually find expression in student behavior than the more ambiguous "Behave in class" or "Do what you are told."

2. *It is more effective to tell students what to do than what not to do.* This accentuation of the positive would, for example, find expression in rules about taking turns, or talking over disagreements, or working quietly, rather than in rules directing students not to jump in, or not to fight, or not to speak out.

3. *Rules should be communicated in such a way that students can memorize them.* Depending on the age of the students, and the complexity and difficulty of enactment of the rules the teacher is presenting, memorization aides may include (1) keeping the rules short; (2) keeping the rules few in number; (3) repeating your presentation of the rules several times; and (4) posting the rules in written form where they can be seen readily.

4. *Rule adherence is likely to be more effective when students have had a substantial role in their development, modification, and implementation.* This sense of participation may be brought about by (1) explicit student involvement in rule development; (2) thorough discussion of rules with the entire class; (3) having selected students explain to the class the

specific meaning of each rule; and (4) student role play of the behaviors identified by the rule.

5. *Rules should be developed at the start of the school year, before other less useful and less explicit rules emerge.* They must be fair, reasonable, and within the student's capacity to follow them; all members of the class should be able to understand them; and they should be applied equally and evenly to all class members.

OBSERVING AND RECORDING BEHAVIOR

The teacher and the class have set behavioral goals and the rules that are the paths to be followed in getting there. The teacher's attention can now turn to the particular students displaying those aggressive, disruptive, rule-breaking, or goal-avoiding behaviors he or she wishes to modify. In doing so, the first task is to identify as concretely as possible the specific behaviors to be changed. Stated otherwise, the beginning stages of behavior modification include specifying (1) desirable or appropriate behaviors (goal behaviors), (2) behavioral means to reach these goals (rule behaviors), and (3) the undesirable or inappropriate behaviors to be altered. This last stage—and here, inappropriate means aggressive—ideally proceeds by means of systematic observation and recording. A number of purposes are served by this process.

First, systematic observation and recording are ways to identify not only undesirable behaviors but also the rate or frequency of such behaviors. This establishment of a base rate permits the teacher to compare later behavior with the base rate to determine whether the behavior is remaining constant, increasing in frequency, or decreasing. This monitoring of change in behavior over time is, then, the second purpose of systematic observation and recording. Finally, the third purpose is to evaluate the success or failure of the completed intervention. At all three stages of this process—establishment of a base rate, monitoring, evaluation of outcome—it is crucial that observation and recording be conducted in a systematic manner. Many authorities on classroom contingency management have commented that teachers' guesses regarding the rate or frequency of a student's aggressive, disruptive, or acting-out behavior are often erroneously high. It is as if a small number of seriously disruptive behaviors by a student can lead to a teacher's global impression of the student as a troublemaker or as chronically aggressive, an impression or label that often obscures the fact that most of the time that youngster is engaged in appropriate behaviors. Thus, it is crucial to obtain an accurate accounting of how often or how long the student engages in problematic behaviors.

Who, then shall the observer be? The teacher must face daily, and try to teach, a full classroom of youngsters, not just those few who sometimes behave aggressively. But the contingency management literature contains numerous examples of teachers as observer—recorders; also teacher aides, parents, peers, and the target youngsters themselves can serve. For whoever serves in this capacity, the task is greatly facilitated when material has been prepared explicitly for such purposes. Recording sheets, special classroom behavior charts, wrist counters, and other similar means are good aids to observer–recorders in systematically identifying and noting representative samples of the frequency or rate of students' inappropriate behaviors (see Jackson, Della-Piana, & Sloane, 1975; Morris, 1976; Sarason et al., 1972; Walker, 1979).

We close our discussion of this phase of the contingency management process with an excerpt from Walker (1979) that reiterates the all-important theme that throughout the process, the teacher should think and act in strictly behavioral terms. Commenting on the observation–recording process, Walker (1979) notes:

> Pinpointing requires attention to the overt features of child behavior. Classroom behaviors that are capable of being pinpointed are characterized by being: (1) controllable, (2) repeatable, (3) containing movement, (4) possessing a starting and ending point. Instances and noninstances of classroom behaviors that qualify as behavioral pinpoints are listed below:
>
> Instances of Good Pinpoints
> 1. Argues
> 2. Steals
> 3. Does not comply with directions
> 4. Out of seat
> 5. Talks out
> 6. Has temper tantrums
> 7. Hits peers
> 8. Looks away from assigned tasks
>
> Noninstances of Good Pinpoints
> 1. Hyperactive
> 2. Lazy
> 3. Belligerent
> 4. Angry
> 5. Hostile
> 6. Frustrated
> 7. Unmotivated (p. 55)

IDENTIFYING POSITIVE REINFORCERS

At this point in the contingency management sequence, the teacher is aware of goals, rules, and specific inappropriate behaviors. Our purpose is to replace these inappropriate behaviors with appropriate ones by means of skilled management of contingencies. One means for doing this is to present positive reinforcement to the student following, and contingent upon, the occurrence of an instance of appropriate behavior. Before discussing procedures for presenting positive reinforcers we must first consider the process of identifying—both for a particular youngster and for youngsters in general—just what events may in fact function as positive reinforcers.

Classroom contingency managers have worked successfully with four types of positive reinforcers: material, social, activity, and token. *Material* or tangible reinforcers are desirable goods or objects presented to the individual contingent upon his or her enactment of appropriate behaviors. One especially important subcategory of material reinforcement, primary reinforcement, occurs when the contingent event presented satisfies a biological need. Food is one such primary reinforcer.

Social reinforcers, most often expressed in the form of attention, praise, or approval, are a particularly powerful and frequent classroom reinforcer. Both anecdotal evidence and extensive experimental research testify to the potency of teacher-dispensed social reinforcement in influencing a broad array of personal inter personal, and academic student behaviors.

Activity reinforcers are those events the youngster chooses to engage in when given a choice of several different activities. For example, many youngsters will choose to watch television rather than complete their homework. The parent wishing to use this activity reinforcer information will tell the youngster that he or she may watch television for a given time period contingent upon the prior completion of the homework. Stated otherwise, the opportunity to perform a high-probability behavior (given free choice) can be used as a reinforcer for a lower-probability behavior.

Token reinforcers, usually employed when more easily implemented social reinforcers prove insufficient, are symbolic items or currency (chips, stars, points, etc.) provided to the youngster contingent upon the performance of appropriate or desirable behaviors. Tokens thus obtained are exchangeable for a wide range of material or activity reinforcers. The system by which specific numbers of tokens are contingently gained (or lost), and the procedures by which they may be exchanged for the backup material or activity reinforcers, is called a "token economy."

In making decisions about which type of reinforcer to employ with a given youngster, the teacher should keep in mind that social reinforcement (e.g., teacher attention, praise, approval) is easiest to implement on a continuing basis, is most likely to lead to enduring behavior change, and is thus probably the type of reinforcement the teacher will wish to use most frequently. Unfortunately, in the initial stages of a behavior-change effort, especially when aggressive, disruptive, and other inappropriate behaviors are likely being rewarded by the social reinforcement of teacher and peer attention, heavier reliance on material and activity reinforcers will likely be more appropriate.

Alternatively, a token reinforcement system may prove most effective as the initial reinforcement strategy. Youngsters' reinforcement preferences change over time, and teachers' views of the appropriate reward value of desirable behaviors also change; both factors are easily reflected in token-level adjustments. For these reasons, and because token systems are both easily administered and effective, the skilled contingency manager should be acquainted with the full range of token economy procedures (Ayllon & Azrin, 1968; Christopherson, Arnold, Hill, & Quilitch, 1972; Kazdin, 1975; Morris, 1976; Walker, Hops, & Fiegenbaum, 1976). Again, however, it is crucial to remember that with but a few exceptions, reliance on material, activity, or token reinforcement must eventually give way to reliance upon social reinforcement that is more like real life.

Table 4.1, excerpted from Safer and Allen (1976), lists specific examples of commonly used materials (edible and nonedible), social, activity, and token reinforcers.

Given this wide yet incomplete array of several types of potential reinforcers, and the fact that almost any event may serve as a reinforcer for one individual but not another, how may the teacher or others decide which reinforcer(s) are best to use with a particular youngster at a given time? Most simply, the youngster can be asked which events he or she would like best. Often, however, this approach will not be sufficient because youngsters do not usually know the range of reinforcers available to them or, if they do, may discount the possibility that a reinforcers will be forthcoming. When this is the case, other reinforcement identification procedures must be employed. Carr (1981) and others have reported three procedures which typically have been used for this purpose.

Observing Effects

The teacher can often make an accurate determination as to whether a given event is functioning as a reinforcer by carefully observing its

TABLE 4.1. Commonly Used Reinforcers

Edible	Nonedible	Social	Activity	Token points
Gum	Balloons	Attention	Gym time	(For
Candy	Clothes	Public praise	Shop time	general
M & M's	Scout uniform	Posting work in	Library time	exchange)
Popcorn	Shoes, etc.	school or at	Driver's license	
Cracker Jacks	Toys (dolls, cars)	home	Movies	
Sodas	Sports-related	Approval	Concerts (folk,	
Cakes	items	Access to	rock, ballet)	
Pies	Baseball cards	privilege areas	Field trips	
Ice cream	Baseball	(e.g., black-	Hobbies	
Hamburgers	Sports	board, lavatory,	Theater	
Nuts	equipment	parent's office,	Ballet	
Raisins	Records	den, TV room)	Sports teams	
	Music equipment	Time off from	Camping	
	Car parts (also	school	Travel	
	motorcyle, etc.,	Hours for out-of-	Day trips	
	parts)	house	Overnight trips	
	Motorcycle, mini-	Private areas		
	bike, bicycle	Private times		
	Furnishings for	TV privileges		
	room (TV,	Program choice		
	posters, black	Time watching		
	lights, dolls)	Dinner out		
	Telephone	Dinnertime choice		
		Friend's privileges		
		In house, at		
		dinner		
		Overnight		
		Bedtime		
		Bath choices		
		Parties		
		Time with one		
		parent		
		Special work		
		Collecting		
		papers		
		Run recorders		
		Carrying		
		messages		
		Telephone		
		privilege		
		Hair length		
		Clothing choice		

Note. From Safer and Allen (1976, pp. 154–155). Copyright 1976 University Park Press. Reprinted by permission.

impact on the youngster. If the youngster (1) asks that the event be repeated; (2) seems happy during the event's occurrence; (3) seems unhappy when the event ends; or (4) will work in order to earn the event, the chances are good that the event is a positive reinforcer and that it can be contingently provided to strengthen appropriate, nonaggressive behaviors.

Observing Choices

As we noted earlier in connection with activity reinforcers, when a youngster is free to choose among several equally available activities, which one he or she chooses, and how long he or she engages in the chosen activity are both readily observed. These are youngster-identified positive reinforcers.

Questionnaires

A small number of questionnaires exist that have been used effectively in identifying positive reinforcers. Tharp and Wetzel's (1969) Mediation-Reinforcer Incomplete Blank is one example. It consists of a series of incomplete sentences that the youngster must complete by specifying particular reinforcers—for example, "The thing I like to do best with my mother/father is . . ." or "I will do almost anything to get . . ."[1] The response format of this questionnaire also asks the youngster to indicate his or her sense of the potency of the reinforcer written in for each item. Thus, this measure provides a self-report of which events are reinforcing for the youngster, when delivered or mediated by whom, as well as the youngster's perception of just how reinforcing each event is.

An instrument for identifying positive reinforcers that is especially appropriate for younger children and children with limited verbal abilities is Homme's (1971) Reinforcing Event Menu. This measure is made up of a collection of pictures portraying a variety of material and activity reinforcers, as well as pictures of a number of potential reinforcement mediators. The youngster's task is to select from the events pictured those for which he or she would most like to work.

This process of identifying positive reinforcers completes the series of preparatory steps a teacher or other contingency manager must undertake before actually presenting positive reinforcers in response to appropriate behaviors.

PRESENTING POSITIVE REINFORCERS

The basic principle of contingency management is that the presentation of a reinforcing event, contingent upon the occurrence of a given behavior, will function to increase the likelihood of the reoccurrence of that behavior. Research has demonstrated a substantial number of factors that influence the success of reinforcement, and thus should be reflected in its presentation when seeking to increase appropriate behaviors.

Being Contingent

First although this rule for reinforcer presentations may seem obvious, it is a crucial rule that is sometimes forgotten or inadequately implemented. The connection between the desirable behavior and the subsequent provision of reward should be made clear and explicit to the youngster. As is true for all aspects of a contingency management effort, this description should be behaviorally specific, that is, the connection between particular behavioral acts and reinforcement made clear. Behaviorally ambiguous comments about "good behavior," "being a good boy," "being well behaved," or the like will not serve.

Reinforcing Immediately

Related to the communication of the behavior reinforcement contingency, the more immediately the presentation of reinforcement follows the desirable behavior, the more likely is its effectiveness. Not only will rapid reinforcement augment the message that the immediately preceding behavior is desirable, but delayed reinforcer presentation runs the risk that a sequence will occur of (1) desirable behavior, (2) undesirable behavior, (3) reinforcement intended for (1) which in actuality reinforces (2).

Reinforcing Consistently

The effects of positive reinforcement on altering behavior are usually gradual, not dramatic. Behavior can be slowly strengthened over time. Positive reinforcement must be presented consistently, not only should the teacher be consistent, but the teacher must try to ensure that all reinforcement delivery efforts are matched by similar efforts from as many other important persons in the youngster's life as possible. Concretely, this means that when the youngster enacts the behavior to be reinforced, in school in the presence of other teachers, at home in the presence of parents or siblings, or at play in the presence of peers, such reinforcement ideally will be forthcoming.

Frequency of Reinforcement

When first trying to establish a new, appropriate behavior, the teacher should seek to reinforce all or almost all instances of that behavior. This high frequency of reinforcement is necessary at first to establish the behavior in the individual's behavioral repertoire. Once it seems this has happened, the teacher may thin the reinforcement schedule, decreasing the presentation of reinforcement so that only some of the youngster's desirable behaviors are followed by reinforcement. This partial reinforcement strategy is an important contribution to the continued likelihood that the appropriate behavior will endure because such a schedule more closely parallels the sometimes-reinforced-sometimes-not reaction the youngster's appropriate behavior will elicit in other settings. A teacher's partial reinforcement of a youngster's appropriate behaviors may be on a fixed time schedule (e.g., at the end of each class), on a fixed number of responses schedule (e.g., every fifth instance of the appropriate behavior), or on variable time or number of response schedules. In any event, the basic strategy for reinforcement frequency remains—a rich level for initial learning and partial reinforcement to sustain performance.

Amount of Reinforcement

We have begun to distinguish between learning—that is, acquiring knowledge about how to perform new behaviors—and performance, that is, using these behaviors. The amount of reinforcement provided influences performance much more than learning. Youngsters will learn new, appropriate behaviors just about as fast for a small reward as for a large one, but they are more likely to perform the behaviors on a continuing basis when large rewards are involved. Yet, rewards can be too large, causing a satiation effect in which the youngster loses interest in seeking the given reinforcement because it is "too much of a good thing." Or, rewards can be too small—too little time on the playground, too few tokens, too thin a social reinforcement schedule. The optimal amount can be determined empirically. If a youngster has worked energetically in the past to obtain a particular reinforcer but gradually slacks off and seems to lose interest in obtaining it, a satiation effect has probably occurred and the amount of reinforcement should be reduced. On the other hand, if a youngster seems unwilling to work for a reinforcer you believe he or she desires, try giving it once or twice for free, that is, not contingent on a specific desirable behavior. If the child seems to enjoy the reinforcer and even wishes more of the same, the amount you had been using may have been too small. Increase the amount, make it contingent, and observe whether it is yielding the desired effect. If so, the amount of reinforcement you are offering is inappropriate.

Variety of Reinforcers

Another type of reinforcement satiation occurs when the teacher uses the same approving phrase or other reward over and over again. Youngsters may perceive such reinforcement as taking on a mechanized quality; thus they may thus lose interest in or responsiveness to it. By varying the content of the reinforcer, the teacher can maintain its potency. Thus, instead of repeating "nice job" four or five times, using a mix of comments — "I'm really proud of you" or "You're certainly doing fine" or "Well done" — is more likely to yield a sustained effect.

Pairing with Praise

Social reinforcement is most germane to enduring behavior change, though there are circumstances under which an emphasis upon material, activity, or token reinforcers is (at least initially) more appropriate. To aid in the desired movement toward social reinforcement, the teacher should try to pair all presentations of material, activity, or token reward with some expression of social reinforcement: an approving comment, a pat on the back, a wink, a smile, and so forth. A major benefit of this tactic is noted by Walker (1979):

> By virtue of being consistently paired with reinforcement delivery, praise can take on the reinforcing properties of the actual reinforcer(s) used. This is especially important since teacher praise is not always initially effective with many deviant children. By systematically increasing the incentive value of praise through pairing, the teacher is in a position to gradually reduce the frequency of [material, activity, or token] reinforcement and to substitute praise. After systematic pairing, the teacher's praise may be much more effective in maintaining the child's appropriate behavior. (p. 108)

Shaping New Behaviors

Reinforcement cannot be presented as contingent upon new behaviors when such behaviors are not part of the youngster's behavioral repertoire. A child cannot be rewarded for talking over disputes with other students at the proper frequency, amount, consistency, and so forth, if he or she never does so. Yet the teacher is not doomed here to perpetual waiting, reinforcers at the ready, for nonemergent desirable behaviors; approximations to such desirable negotiating behaviors, even remote approximations, can be positively reinforced. Looking at the other disputant, walking towards him or her, discussing an irrelevant (to the dispute) topic are all reinforcible steps in the direction of the ultimately desired behaviors. By this process of reinforcing behaviors successively closer to the final target behavior, coupled with successive withdrawal of such reinforcement for less good approximations, the behavior-change process can proceed in a stepwise fashion in which youngsters' behaviors are systematically shaped into ever-better approximations to the final target behavior.

These aforementioned rules for maximizing the effectiveness of the presentation of positive reinforcement are all essentially remedial in nature. They are efforts to substitute appropriate, prosocial behaviors for aggressive, disruptive, or antisocial behaviors which have already been displayed. It is also worth noting, however that the presentation of positive reinforcement may be used for preventive purposes. Sarason et al. (1972) urge teachers to openly present positive reinforcement to specific youngsters in such a manner that the entire class is aware of it. They comment:

> Positive reinforcement for productive activity for the whole group is a powerful preventive technique. It can eliminate or reduce the great majority of behavior problems in classrooms. Try to praise the children who are paying attention. Attend to those who are sitting in their seats, doing their work in a nondisruptive manner. "That's right, John, you're doing a good job." "You watched the board all the time I was presenting the problem. That's paying attention." . . . These responses not only reinforce the child to whom they are directed, but they also help to provide the rest of the class with an explicit idea of what you mean by paying attention and working hard. Young children, especially . . . learn to model their actions after the positive examples established and noted by the teacher. (p. 18)

Additional sources of information about the experimental evidence in support of these procedures for contingency management follow. Especially comprehensive reviews include Baer, Blount, Detrick, and Stokes (1987); Bandura (1969); Gambrill (1977); Kazdin (1977, 1987,

1989); Kerr, Strain, and Ragland (1982); Nafpaltitis, Mayer, and Butterworth (1985); O'Leary and O'Leary (1976, 1980); Pfiffner, Rosen, and O'Leary (1985); Reid and Patterson (1991), and Walker (1979).

Individual studies that are particularly instructive for using these procedures with aggressive or disruptive youngsters are those of Adams (1973); Becker, Madsen, Arnold, and Thomas (1967); Buys (1972); Hall, Panyan, Rabon, and Broden (1968); Kirschner and Levin (1975); Pinkston, Reese, LeBlanc, and Baer (1973), Sewell, McCoy, and Sewell (1973), and Ward and Baker (1968).

REMOVING POSITIVE REINFORCERS

The teacher's behavior modification goal with youngsters displaying aggressive behaviors is, in a general sense, twofold. Both sides of the behavioral coin — appropriate and inappropriate, prosocial and antisocial, desirable and undesirable — must be attended to. In a proper behavior-change effort, procedures are simultaneously or sequentially employed to reduce and eliminate the inappropriate, antisocial, or undesirable components of the youngster's behavioral repertoire, and to increase the quality and frequency of appropriate, prosocial, or desirable components. This latter task is served primarily by the contingent presentation of positive reinforcement. Conversely, the contingent removal of positive reinforcement in response to aggressive, disruptive, or similar behaviors is the major behavior modification strategy for reducing or eliminating such behaviors. Therefore, in conjunction with the procedures discussed previously for presenting positive reinforcement, the teacher should also simultaneously or consecutively employ one or more of the three positive-reinforcer-removing techniques we now examine.

EXTINCTION

Knowing When to Use Extinction

Extinction is the withdrawal or removal of positive reinforcement for aggressive or other undesirable behaviors that have been either deliberately or inadvertently reinforced in the past. It is the procedure of choice with milder forms of aggression, such as threats, swearing, or other forms of verbal aggression, or with low-amplitude physical aggression. More generally, extinction should be used when other individuals are not in any serious physical danger from the aggression being displayed. Determining the appropriateness of extinction is, of course, in part a function of each teacher's tolerance for deviance and his or her classroom management philosophy, but extinction is often used by teachers and classroom peers who are trying to ignore some ongoing inappropriate behavior. Each teacher will have to decide which undesirable behaviors can be safely ignored. Taking a conservative stance, Walker (1979) suggests that extinction "should be applied only to those inappropriate behaviors that are minimally disruptive to class-room atmosphere" (p. 40). Others are somewhat more liberal in its application—for example, Carr (1981). In any event, it is clear that the first step in applying extinction is knowing when to use it.

It is also clear that attempts to reduce inappropriate behavior by reinforcement withdrawal should always be accompanied by efforts to increase appropriate behaviors by providing reinforcement. This com-bination will succeed especially well when the appropriate and inap-propriate behaviors involved are opposite, or at least incompatible with one another. For example, reward in-seat behavior, ignore out-of-seat behavior; reward talking at a conversational level, ignore yelling.

Using essentially the same observation and recording procedures described earlier (see pp. 80–81) in conjunction with the identification of positive reinforcers maintaining appropriate behaviors, the teacher should discern what the youngster is working for, what are his or her payoffs, and what are the reinforcers being sought or earned by ag-gression, disruptiveness, and similar behaviors. Very often the answer will be attention. Laughing, looking, staring, yelling at, talking to, or turning toward are common teacher and peer reactions to a young-ster's aggression. The withdrawal of such positive social reinforcement by ignoring the behaviors, by turning away, by not yelling or talking or laughing at the perpetrator are the behaviors that would constitute extinction. Ignoring someone whom you would normally attend to is itself a talent, as the next extinction rule illustrates.

Carr (1981) has suggested three useful guidelines for ignoring low-level aggressive behaviors:

1. *Do not comment to the child that you are ignoring him or her.* Long (or even short) explanations provided to youngsters about why others are going to stop paying attention to certain behaviors provide just the type of social reinforcement that in extinction must be withdrawn. Such explanations are to be avoided.

2. *Do not look away suddenly when the child behaves aggressively.* Jerk-ing one's head away suddenly so as not to see the continuation of the aggressive behavior, or any other such abrupt behavior by the teacher, may also communicate the message "I really noticed and was impelled

to action by your behavior." As Carr (1981) recommends, "It is best to ignore the behavior by reacting to it in a matter of fact way by continuing natural ongoing activities" (p. 38).

3. *Do protect the victims of aggression.* If one youngster actually strikes another, the teacher must intervene to protect the victim. One may do so without subverting the extinction effort by providing the victim with attention, concern, and interest, and by ignoring the perpetrator of the aggression.

Using Extinction Consistently

As was true for the provision of reinforcement, its removal must be consistent if its intended effects are to be forthcoming. In a classroom, this rule of consistency means both that the teacher and classmates must act in concert, and that the teacher must be consistent across time. In a school, consistency means that if possible, all teachers having significant contact with a youngster must strive to ignore the same inappropriate behaviors. In addition, to avoid letting a youngster think, "I can't act up here, but I can out there" parent conferences should be held to bring parents, siblings, and other significant real world figures into the extinction effort. As Karoly (1980) notes, when consistency of non-attending is not reached, the aggressive behavior will be intermittently or partially reinforced, a circumstance that would lead to its becoming highly resistant to extinction.

Using Extinction Long Enough

Aggressive behaviors often have a long history of positive reinforcement and, especially if much of that history is one of intermittent reinforcement, efforts to undo it must be sustained. Persistence in this regard will, however, usually succeed. Carr (1981) suggests that within a week, clear reductions in aggressive behavior should be observable. There are, however, two possibly misleading events to keep in mind when judging the effectiveness of extinction efforts. The first is known as the *extinction burst.* When extinction is first introduced, it is not uncommon for the rate or intensity of the aggressive behavior to first increase sharply before it begins its more gradual decline toward a zero level. It is important that the teacher not get discouraged during this short detour in direction. Its meaning, in fact, is that the extinction is beginning to work. The second is *spontaneous recovery.* On occasion, inappropriate behaviors which have been successfully extinguished will reappear, for reasons that are difficult to determine. Like the extinction burst, this recovery phenomenon is transitory, and will disappear if the teacher persists in the extinction effort.

The effectiveness of extinction in modifying inappropriate or undesirable behaviors in a classroom context has been demonstrated by many investigators, including Brown and Elliott (1965); Carlson and Lahey (1988); Gilliam, Stough, and Fad (1991); Iwata (1987); Jones and Miller (1974); Kanfer and Goldstein (1991); Madsen, Becker, and Thomas (1968); Nemeroff and Karoly (1991); Wahler, Winkel, Peterson, and Morrison (1965); and Ward and Baker (1968).

TIME-OUT

Time-out is a removal from positive reinforcement; a youngster who engages in aggressive or other inappropriate behaviors is physically removed from all sources of reinforcement for a specified time period. As with extinction, the purpose of time-out is to reduce the undesirable behavior which immediately precedes it, and on which its use is contingent. It differs from extinction in that extinction involves removing reinforcement from the person, whereas time-out usually involves removing the person from the reinforcing situation. In classroom practice, time out has typically taken three forms. *Isolation time-out,* the most common form, requires that the youngster be physically removed from the classroom to a time-out room. *Exclusion time-out* is somewhat less restrictive, but also involves physically removing the youngster from sources of reinforcement. Here the youngster is required to go to a corner of the classroom, and perhaps to sit in a "quiet chair" (Firestone, 1976), sometimes also behind a screen. The youngster is not removed from the classroom, but is excluded from classroom activities for a specific time period. *Nonexclusion time-out* (also called contingent observation), the least restrictive time-out variant, requires the youngster to "sit and watch" on the periphery of classroom activities, to observe the appropriate behaviors of other youngsters. It is a variant which, in a sense, combines time-out with modeling opportunities (see p. 107). Its essence is to exclude the youngster from a participant role for a specified time period, while leaving intact the opportunity to function as an observer.

Knowing When to Use Time-Out

Extinction was the recommended procedure for those aggressive or otherwise undesirable behaviors that could be safely ignored. Behaviors

that are potentially injurious to other youngsters require a more active teacher response, possibly time-out. Yet, for many youngsters at
the upper junior high school and high school levels, physically removing students is often neither wise, appropriate, nor even possible. For
such youngsters, procedures other than extinction or time-out must be
employed. Thus, to reflect both the potential injuriousness of the youngster's behavior and the youngster's age and associated physical status,
time-out is recommended as the technique of choice for youngsters aged
2 to 12 who are displaying high rates of severely aggressive behavior
that is potentially dangerous to others. It is also the best procedure for
less severe forms of aggression, when the combination of extinction
and positive reinforcement for milder levels of aggression has been
attempted and has failed.

As with providing positive reinforcement, time-out should be used
in tandem. When possible, the behaviors positively reinforced should
be opposite to, or at least incompatible with, those for which the time
out procedure is instituted. Furthermore, there is an additional basis
for recommending the combined use of these two techniques. As Carr
(1981) observes:

> Although one important reason for using positive reinforcement is to
> strengthen nonaggressive behaviors to the point where they replace ag-
> gressive behaviors, there is a second reason for using reinforcement proce-
> dures. If extensive use of positive reinforcement is made, then time out
> will become all the more aversive since it would involve the temporary
> termination of a rich diversity of positive reinforcers. In this sense, then,
> the use of positive reinforcement helps to enhance the effectiveness of
> the time-out procedure. (pp. 41–42)

Arranging a Time-Out Setting

The general principles of an isolation time out arrangement readily
carry over to both exclusion and nonexclusion time-out environments.
Essentially, two general principles are involved; the first concerns the
youngster's health and safety. The time-out setting should be a small,
well-lit, and well-ventilated room that provides a place for the youngster
to sit. The second principle reflects the fact that the main feature of
this procedure is the time-out it provides from positive reinforcement.
It must be a boring environment, with all reinforcers removed. There
should be no attractive or distracting objects or opportunities: no toys,
television, radio, books, posters, people, windows to look out, sound
sources to overhear, or other obvious or not-so-obvious potential reinforcers. A barren, isolation area is the best time-out environment.

Placing a Youngster in Time-Out

A number of actions may be taken by the teacher when initiating time-out that serve to increase the likelihood of its effectiveness. As with the rapid presentation of positive reinforcement that is contingent upon appropriate behaviors, time-out is optimally instituted immediately following the aggressive or other behaviors you are seeking to modify. Having explained earlier to the class what time-out meant, as well as when and why it would be used, the teacher should implement it in a matter of fact manner following undesirable behavior, that is, in a way that minimizes the social reinforcement of the aggression. Concretely, this means placing the youngster in time-out without a lengthy explanation, but with a brief, description of his or her precipitating behaviors. This placement process is best conducted without anger by the teacher, and without (when possible) having to use physical means for moving the youngster from the classroom to the time-out room.

Consistent with seeking to minimize reinforcement of aggression during this process, it is also best if the distance between classroom and time-out room is small — the shorter the distance, the shorter the transportation time, and the less opportunity for inadvertent social reinforcement by the teacher. In addition to these considerations, the effectiveness of time-out is further enhanced by its consistent application when appropriate, by the same teacher on other occasions as well as by other teachers. Immediacy, consistency, and the various actions aimed at minimizing teacher presentation of reinforcement following inappropriate behavior each function to augment the behavior-change effectiveness of time-out.

Maintaining a Youngster in Time-Out

The skilled contingency manager must deal with two questions during a youngster's period in time-out: "What is he or she doing?" and "For how long should time-out last?" Answering the first question by teacher monitoring makes certain that the time out experience is not in fact functioning as a pleasant, positively reinforcing one for a given youngster. For example, rather than serve as a removal from positive reinforcement, time-out may in reality be a removal from an aversive situation (negative reinforcement) if the teacher institutes it at a time when a youngster is in an unpleasant situation from which he or she would prefer to escape, or if time-out makes it possible to avoid such a situation. Similarly, if monitoring reveals that the youngster is singing or playing enjoyable games, the effectiveness of time-out will be lessened. Unless the situation can be made essentially nonreinforcing, a different behavioral intervention may have to be used.

With regard to the duration of time-out, most of its successful implementations have been from 5 to 20 minutes long, with some clear preference for the shorter periods of this range. When experimenting to find the optimal duration for any given youngster it is best, as White, Nielsen, and Johnson (1972) have shown, to begin with a short duration (e.g., 3 to 5 minutes) and lengthen the time out until an effective span is identified, rather than to successively shorten an initially longer span. This latter approach would, again, risk the possibility of introducing an event experienced as positive reinforcement by the youngster.

Releasing a Youngster from Time-Out

We noted earlier in connection with extinction that the implementation of a withdrawal of positive reinforcement sometimes leads to initial instances — extinction bursts — in which more intense or more frequent aggressiveness appears before it begins to subside. This same pattern is evident with withdrawal from positive reinforcement, that is, time-out. The first few times a youngster is placed in time-out there might be called a *time-out burst* of heightened aggressiveness. These bursts will usually subside, especially if the teacher adds to the duration of the time-out period the same number of minutes that the outburst lasted.

Whether the release of the youngster from time-out is on schedule or is delayed for reasons just specified, the release should be conducted in a matter-of-fact manner and the youngster quickly returned to regular classroom activities. Long explanations or apologies at this time are, once again, tactically erroneous provisions of positive reinforcement that communicate to the youngster that acting out in the classroom will bring him or her a short period of removal from reinforcement and then a probably longer period of undivided teacher attention.

The effectiveness of time-out in substantially reducing or eliminating aggressive or disruptive behaviors has been shown by Allison and Allison (1971); Blechman (1985); Bostow and Bailey (1969); Calhoun and Matherne (1975); Lentz (1988); Mace, Page, Ivancic, and O'Brien (1986); Mayer and Sulzer-Azaroff (1991); Nelson and Rutherford (1983); Drabman and Spitalnik (1973); Patterson, Cobb, and Ray (1973); Patterson and Reid (1973); Vukelich and Hake (1971); Wahler and Fox (1980); Webster (1976); and White et al. (1972).

RESPONSE COST

"Response cost" refers to the removal of previously acquired reinforcers contingent upon the occurrence of inappropriate behaviors. The reinforcers previously acquired and herein contingently removed may have been earned, as when the use of response-cost procedures are a component of a token-reinforcement system, or they may have been simply provided, as is the case with a free-standing no-token-economy response-cost system. In either instance, reinforcers are removed (the cost) wherever previously targeted undesirable behaviors occur (the response). The two other means we have examined for the systematic removal of positive reinforcement, extinction and time-out, have often been insufficient for delinquent or severely aggressive mid- and late-adolescents, even when combined with teacher praise or other reinforcement for appropriate behaviors. In a number of these instances, response-cost procedures, especially when combined with the provision of positive reinforcement (e.g., via a token-economy system) for desirable behaviors, have proven effective. Thus, not only must a teacher's selection of approach be a prescriptive function of target youngster characteristics, but the teacher must also continue, in implementing this approach, to combine its use with tandem procedures for providing positive reinforcement of appropriate behaviors.

We do not detail here the rules for the effective implementation of a token-economy system, as they overlap considerably with rules delineated earlier for the provision of nontoken positive reinforcers (see pp. 86–90), and may be found in Christopherson et al. (1972); Ayllon and Azrin (1968); Kazdin (1975); Morris (1976); and Walker et al. (1976). We do wish to specify, however, those rules for token- or nontoken-reinforcement removal which constitute the essence of the response-cost procedure.

DEFINING INAPPROPRIATE BEHAVIORS

As with every other contingency management procedure, the teacher must think, plan, and act behaviorally. When specifying the inappropriate target behaviors whose occurrence will cost tokens, points, privileges, or other commodities or events, specific overt acts must be delineated, not broader behavioral characterological categories. Thus, "is aggressive" (an observation of character) or "acts aggressively" (an observation of broad behavior) are too vague, but "swears, makes threats, raises voice, raises hands, pushes classmate" are all more useful specifications.

As with every other contingency management procedure, it is requisite that the teacher think, plan, and act behaviorally. When specifying the inappropriate target behaviors whose occurrence will cost tokens, points, privileges, or other commodities or events, specific overt acts must be delineated, not broad behavioral characterological categories. Thus, "is aggressive" (a characterological observation) or "acts aggressively" (a broad behavioral observation) are too vague, but "swears, makes threats, raises voice, raises hands, pushes classmate" are all more useful specifications.

DETERMINING THE COST

Just as the amount, level, or rate of positive reinforcement to be provided contingent upon desirable behaviors must be determined, so must the specific cost—whether such cost is a number of tokens or points, amount of time the television will be kept off, or something else. Cost setting is a crucial determinant of the success or failure of implementing this approach. For example, Carr (1981) notes:

> The magnitude of response cost must be carefully controlled. If fines are too large, bankruptcy will ensue and the child will be unable to purchase any back-up reinforcers. Further, if the child develops too large a deficit, he may adapt an attitude of "what do I have to lose?" and engage in considerable misbehavior. On the other hand, if the fines are too small, the child will be able to negate his loss easily by performing any of a variety of appropriate behaviors. (p. 52)

Yet other aspects of response-cost implementation will make demands on the teacher's skills as a creative economist. The relationship of points or other reinforcers available to earn to those one can lose, the relationship of cost to the severity of the inappropriate behavior, and a host of similar marketing, pricing, and, ultimately, motivational considerations, may come into play and thus require a substantial level of contingency management expertise on the part of the teacher. This is especially true if the teacher is not only the implementer of the response-cost system, but also its originator, planner, and monitor.

Communicating Contingencies

Once the teacher has decided upon the specific token, point, or privilege value of the appropriate and inappropriate behaviors relevant to the effective management of his or her classroom, these values must be communicated to the class. A readily visible reinforcer value list indicating earnings and losses should be drawn up and posted. Table 4.2 is a composite example of such a list, designed to be appropriate at the junior high school level.

Removing Reinforcement

Class members must not only know in advance what earnings and losses are contingent upon what desirable and undesirable behaviors, but each must also have ongoing access to his or her own earnings status. A good example of how this may be accomplished is provided by Walker (1979) who has developed a simple, easily used delivery/feedback system which gives each youngster ongoing cumulative information in-

TABLE 4.2. Behaviors That Earn and Lose Points

Behaviors	Number of points
Earn points	
1. Reading books	5 per page
2. Greeting people appropriately	100 per instance
3. Remaining in seat	100 per 15 minutes
4. Taking notes	250 per 15 minutes
5. Being on time for school	250 per day
6. Being quiet in lunch line	300 per instance
7. Being quiet in cafeteria	300 per instance
8. Displaying appropriate playground behavior	500 per 15 minutes
9. Doing complete homework	1000 per day
10. Getting an A/B/C/D grade	2000/1000/500/250 per grade
11. Talking out disagreements	1000 per instance
Lose points	
1. Greeting people inappropriately	100 per instance
2. Being out of seat inappropriately	150 per instance
3. Being late for school	10 per minute
4. Being noisy in classroom	300 per instance
5. Being noisy in lunch line	300 per instance
6. Being noisy in cafeteria	300 per instance
7. Swearing	500 per instance
8. Cheating	1000 per instance
9. Having incomplete homework	1000 per instance
10. Getting an F grade	1000 per grade
11. Showing physical aggression	1000 per instance
12. Stealing	2500 per instance

dicating (1) when response cost (or earnings) has been applied; (2) to which specific behaviors it was applied; and (3) how many points have been lost (or earned) as a result. In implementing the response cost component of this system, each youngster was given a 4 × 6 inch card once each week. The card, whose content appears in Figure 4.1., was taped to the corner of each youngster's desk.

As the first step in implementing the delivery and feedback of response cost, both the use of the cards and the specific behaviors involved in their use were planned and illustrated for the class. During the week, whenever a given youngster engaged in one of the inappropriate behaviors, the teacher walked to the youngster's desk and, with a special marking pen, placed a dot in the box corresponding to the day of the week and to the particular inappropriate behavior to which the cost was being applied. Consistent with the effort to avoid providing social reinforcement while removing positive reinforcement, teachers concurrently told the youngster which behavior(s) were involved and the number of points lost, but engaged in no other dialogue at that time.

A delivery/feedback card such as the one in Figure 4.1 may be used as part of a response-cost system in which the youngster (1) is simply given a fixed number of points initially and noncontingently; (2) keeps or loses points as a function of his or her behavior during a fixed time period; and (3) is given the opportunity to exchange points remaining for backup material or activity reinforcers at the end of that time period. Alternatively, such means for keeping a youngster posted on his or her point status may also be part of a token economy system in which points must be earned (e.g. Table 4.2) contingent on appropriate behaviors, not awarded initially on a noncontingent basis. When this earn-

Behaviors	Point values	M	T	W	T	F
Out of seat	2	• •				
Talk outs	2	•	• •			
Nonattending	1	• • •	•			
Noncompliance	3		•			
Disturbing others	2	•				
Foul language	4		•			
Fighting	5					

FIGURE 4.1. Response-cost delivery/feedback system. The youngster whose appropriate behaviors are recorded here lost 11 points on Monday and 12 points on Tuesday. From Walker (1979, p. 127). Copyright 1979 Allyn and Bacon. Reprinted by permission.

ing requirement is in effect, a second delivery/feedback card (or the reverse side of the response-cost card) may be used to keep an ongoing record of points earned by each youngster in each (appropriate) behavior category each day.

As was true for extinction and time-out, the best implementation of response cost requires that the teacher be (1) *consistent* in his or her application of it across students and across time; (2) *immediate* in delivering contingent costs as soon as possible after the occurrence of inappropriate behavior; and (3) *impartial and inevitable,* in that an instance of such behavior leads to an instance of response cost almost automatically, with a minimum number of special circumstances, special students, or special exceptions.

A number of investigations have independently demonstrated the effectiveness of response cost procedures — for example, Burchard and Barrera (1972); Carey and Bucker (1981); Christopherson et al. (1972); Kaufman and O'Leary (1972); O'Leary and Becker (1967); O'Leary, Becker, Evans, and Saudargas (1969); Pazulinec, Meyerrose, and Sạjivaj (1983); Rapport, Murphy, and Bailey (1982); Salend and Allen (1985); Walker (1983); and Witt and Elliott (1982).

AVERSIVE STIMULI: PRESENTATION AND REMOVAL

We do not recommend the presentation of aversive stimuli (i.e., punishment) or the removal of aversive stimuli (i.e., negative reinforcement) without some accompanying use of positive reinforcement. Our reasons for this are explained in the following discussion.

Punishment

Punishment is the presentation of an aversive stimulus contingent upon the performance of a given behavior, and is usually intended to decrease the likelihood of future occurrences of that behavior. Two of the major forms that punishment has taken in American classrooms are verbal punishment, that is, reprimands, and physical punishment, such as paddling, spanking, slapping, or other forms of corporal punishment. The effectiveness of these and other forms of punishment in altering inappropriate behaviors such as aggression has been shown to be a function of several factors including:

1. Likelihood of punishment.
2. Consistency of punishment.

3. Immediacy of punishment.
4. Duration of punishment.
5. Severity of punishment.
6. Possibility for escape or avoidance of punishment.
7. Availability of alternate routes to goal.
8. Level of instigation to aggression.
9. Level of reward for aggression.
10. Characteristics of the prohibiting agents.

Punishment is more likely to lead to behavior change the more certain its application, the more consistently and rapidly it is applied, the longer and more intense its quality, the less likely it can be avoided, the more available are alternative means to goal satisfaction, the lower the level of instigation to aggression or reward for aggression, and the more potent as a contingency manager is the prohibiting agent. Thus, there are clearly several determinants of the impact of an aversive stimulus on a youngster's behavior.

But let us assume an instance of these determinants' combining to yield a substantial impact. What, ideally, may we hope that the effect of punishment on aggression or other undesirable behavior will be? A reprimand or a paddling will not teach new behaviors. If the youngster is deficient in the ability to ask rather than take, request rather than command, negotiate rather than strike out, all the scolding, scowling, or spanking possible will not teach the youngster the desirable alternative behaviors. Thus punishment, if used at all, must be combined with efforts to instruct the youngster in those behaviors he or she does not know (e.g., by modeling [see p. 107] or related procedures). When the youngster does possess alternative desirable behaviors, but only in approximate form, punishment may best be combined with shaping (see p. 89) procedures. And, when high-quality appropriate behaviors are possessed by the youngster, but he or she is not displaying them, the use of punishment is optimally combined with any of the other procedures described earlier for the systematic presentation of positive reinforcement. In short, punishment should always be combined with a companion procedure for strengthening appropriate alternative behaviors, whether these behaviors are absent, weak, or merely unused in the youngster's behavioral repertoire.

Our urging grows in particular from the fact that most investigators report the main effect of punishment to be a temporary suppression of inappropriate behaviors. Although we appreciate the potential value of such a temporary suppression to the harried classroom teacher seeking a more manageable classroom environment, it is not uncommon, because of this temporariness, for the teacher to have to institute punishment over and over again to the same youngsters for the same inappropriate behaviors. To recapitulate, we urge that if punishment is used, its use be combined with one or another means for simultaneously teaching desirable behaviors—a recommendation underscored by the common finding that when punishment does succeed in altering behavior, such effects are often temporary.

In part because of this temporariness, but more so for other reasons, a number of contingency management researchers have assumed an antipunishment stance, seeing little place for it in the contemporary classroom. This view responds to punishment research demonstrating such undesirable side effects of punishment as withdrawal from social contact, counteraggression toward the punisher, modeling of punishing behavior, disruption of social relationships, failure of effects to generalize, selective avoidance (refraining from inappropriate behaviors only when under surveillance), and stigmatizing labeling effects (Azrin & Holz, 1966; Bandura, 1973).

An alternative, propunishment view does exist. It is less widespread and more controversial but, as with the view of the investigators just cited, it seeks to make its case based upon empirical evidence. Thus, it is held that there are numerous favorable effects of punishment: rapid and dependable reduction of inappropriate behaviors, the consequent opening up of new sources of positive reinforcement, the possibility of complete suppression of inappropriate behaviors, increased social and emotional behavior, imitation and discrimination learning, and other potential positive side effects (Axelrod & Apsche, 1982; Newsom, Favell, & Rincover, 1982; Van Houten, 1982).

The evidence is clearly not all in. Complete data on which punishers should be used with which youngsters under which circumstances are not available. Presently, decisions regarding the classroom use of aversive stimuli to alter inappropriate behaviors must derive from partial data and from each teacher's carefully considered ethical beliefs regarding the relative costs and benefits of employing punishment procedures. Our own weighing of relevant data and ethical considerations leads to our stance favoring the selective use of verbal punishment techniques in classrooms, and our rejecting under all circumstances the use of corporal punishment or similar physical punishment techniques.

Verbal Reprimands

Though results are mixed, the preponderance of research demonstrates that punishment in the form of verbal reprimands is an effective means for reducing disruptive classroom behavior (Jones & Miller, 1974), littering (Risley, 1977), object throwing (Sajwaj, Culver, Hall, & Lehr, 1972), physical aggression (Hall et al., 1971), and other acting-out behaviors (O'Leary, Kaufman, Kass, & Drabman, 1970; Sallis, 1983; Sandler & Steele, 1991; Van Houten & Daley, 1983; Van Houten, Nau, McKenzie-Keating, Sameoto, & Colavecchia, 1982; and Woolridge & Richman, 1985). These and other relevant studies also indicate, beyond overall effectiveness, that reprimands are most potent when the teacher is physically close to the target youngster, clearly specifies in behavioral terms the inappropriate behavior being reprimanded, maintains eye contact with the youngster, uses a firm voice, and firmly grasps the youngster while delivering the reprimand. Finally, White et al. (1972) and Forehand, Roberts, Dolays, Hobbs, and Resick (1976) each compared reprimands to other commonly employed forms of punishment and found reprimands to be superior in effectiveness.

Our position favoring the selective use of teacher reprimands rests jointly on our understanding of the foregoing research findings combined with our cost/benefit belief that such procedures not only have a high likelihood of being effective, but also a low likelihood of being injurious, especially when combined, as we and others have repeatedly urged, with one or another means for presenting positive reinforcement for appropriate behaviors. In this latter regard, both White (1975) and Thomas, Presland, Grant, and Gynn (1978) have independently shown that teachers deliver an average of 0.5 reprimands per minute in both elementary and junior high schools, a rate which substantially exceeds, in all grade levels beyond grade two, their rate of offering praise to students for appropriate behaviors. In other words, teachers now reprimand students at rates which are absolutely very high, and far too infrequently do they accompany such reprimands by social reinforcement for desirable behaviors. We urge a change in this regard.

Corporal Punishment

Newsom et al. (1982) speculate that physically painful punishment that succeeds in altering inappropriate behaviors may be, all in all less injurious and more helpful to a youngster than nonphysically painful but less effective alternatives. We are given pause by their speculation. Nevertheless, we know of no empirical evidence bearing upon it and take a stance opposed to corporal punishment in school (or any other) settings. As Axelrod and Apsche (1982) encourage, our guiding ethical principle is to encourage "the implementation of the least drastic alternative which has a reasonable probability of success" (p. 16). Given the substantial number of demonstrations of effectiveness of procedures involving the presentation of positive reinforcers, the similarly strong results bearing on techniques for removing such reinforcement, the evidence regarding verbal punishment, and the paucity of research evaluating the effectiveness of corporal punishment, we see no place for it in the domain of effective classroom management.

Yet 28 of America's 50 states, representing 51% of America's school children, permit corporal punishment; its school and community advocates seem to be loud, numerous, and growing in numbers. Is it, as Hagebak (1979) darkly suggests, that physically punitive teachers should ask themselves "whether they tend to interpret classroom problems as a personal threat, whether they inflict punishment to protect their self-esteem, whether they retaliate rather than consider the causes of disruptive behavior objectively, and whether they derive sexual satisfaction from inflicting physical punishment" (p. 112)? Or, recalling our definition of negative reinforcement, is teacher use and reuse of corporal punishment a simple function of the fact that it intermittently succeeds in reducing or eliminating the student disruptiveness, aggression, or other behavior experienced as aversive by the teacher?

Whatever motivations and reinforcements have sustained its use, corporal punishment — as is true of all means of punishment — fails to yield a sustained suppression of inappropriate behaviors; it increases the likelihood that the youngster will behave aggressively in other settings (Hyman, 1978; Maurer, 1974; Welsh, 1978), and makes no contribution at all to the development of new, appropriate behaviors. We feel strongly that one's behavior as a classroom teacher must be responsive ethically to such accumulated empirical evidence. The science of behavior modification must replace the folklore of procorporal punishment beliefs.

Negative Reinforcement

Negative reinforcement is the final contingency management procedure we wish to consider, and that will be brief. Recall that negative reinforcement is the removal of aversive stimuli contingent upon the occurrence of desirable behaviors. Negative reinforcement has seldom been used to systematically modify behavior in classrooms. The major exception to this is the manner in which youngsters may be contingently released from time-out (an aversive environment), depending upon such desirable behaviors as quietness and calmness, because such release serves as negative reinforcement for these behaviors. Unfortunately, negative reinforcement often proves important in a classroom context in a less constructive way. Consider a teacher–student interaction in which the student behaves disruptively (shouts, swears, fights), the teacher responds with anger and physical punishment toward the youngster, and the punishment brings about a (temporary) suppression of the youngster's disruptiveness. The decrease in student disruptiveness may also be viewed as a decrease in aversive stimulation experienced by the teacher, which functions to negatively reinforce the immediately preceding teacher behaviors, which might, for example, include corporal punishment. The net effect of this sequence is to increase the likelihood that the teacher will use corporal punishment again. Analogous sequences may occur and function to increase the likelihood of other ineffective, inappropriate, or intemperate teacher behaviors.

OTHER BEHAVIOR MODIFICATION PROCEDURES

In addition to the various procedures we have examined for the presentation or removal of positive reinforcement or aversive stimuli, there are a number of behavior modification procedures available for classroom use that do not rely upon the management of contingencies for their apparent effectiveness. In this section we briefly consider these procedures.

Overcorrection

Overcorrection is a type of behavior modification developed by Foxx and Azrin (1973) for that circumstance when extinction, time out, and response cost have either failed or cannot be used, and there are few available appropriate behaviors to reinforce. Overcorrection is a two-part procedure, having both restitutional and positive practice components. The restitutional aspect requires that the target individual return the behavioral setting (e.g., the classroom) to its predisruption status or better. Thus, the objects broken by an angry youngster must be repaired, the classmates struck in anger apologized to, the papers scattered across the room picked up. Further, the positive practice component of overcorrection requires that the disruptive youngster then, in the examples just cited, be made to repair objects broken by others, or apologize to classmates who witnessed the classmate being struck, or clean up the rest of the classroom including areas not messed up by the target youngster. It is clear that the restitution — positive practice requirements may jointly serve both a punitive and an instructional function.

Modeling

Modeling, also known as imitation learning, vicarious learning, and observational learning, is an especially powerful behavior modification procedure. Modeling may teach new behaviors or strengthen or weaken previously learned behaviors. Its effects have been demonstrated across a particularly wide array of target behaviors, including student aggression (Bandura, 1969; Goldstein, Sprafkin, Gershaw, & Klein, 1979; Perry & Furukawa, 1980; Sarason, 1968). Modeling procedures, facilitators, and consequences are examined in depth in Chapter 3, where we discuss ways to teach prosocial behaviors.

Behavioral Rehearsal

With deep roots both in psychodrama and more contemporaneous role playing activities, behavioral rehearsal has become an important behavior modification procedure. In it, appropriate alternative behaviors are enacted by the target individual in a safe, quasiprotected training environment prior to its utilization in real world contexts. Behavioral rehearsal, which is also described in detail in Chapter 3, is often used in conjunction with modeling (which shows what to rehearse) and feedback (regarding how well the rehearsed behavior matches the model's). With both individuals and groups, behavioral rehearsal has been used effectively to teach such alternatives to aggression as assertiveness (Galassi & Galassi, 1977), negotiation (Goldstein & Rosenbaum, 1982), self-control (Novaco, 1975), and a host of other prosocial behaviors (Goldstein et al., 1979).

Contingency Contracting

A contingency contract is a written agreement between a teacher and student. It is a document each signs that specifies, in behavioral terms, desirable student behaviors and their positive, teacher-provided consequences as well as undesirable student behaviors and their contingent undesirable consequences. As Homme (1971) specified in his initial description of this procedure, such contracts will more reliably lead to desirable student behaviors when the contract payoff is immediate; approximations to the desirable behaviors are rewarded; the contract rewards accomplishment rather than obedience; accomplishment precedes reward; the contract is fair, clear, honest, positive, and systematically implemented.

PROCEDURAL COMBINATIONS

It is increasingly the accepted view in both education and psychology that interventions designed to modify overt behavior in personal, interpersonal, or academic realms are best designed and implemented prescriptively (Cronbach & Snow, 1969; Goldstein, 1978; Goldstein & Stein, 1976; Hunt & Sullivan, 1974). This differential or tailored intervention strategy proposes that the modification of behavior will proceed most effectively and efficiently when methods used prescriptively fit the type or intensity of the behaviors to which they are applied. For the most part, the state of prescriptive guidelines is still largely rudimentary, and only approximate prescriptions are now possible. Such prescriptions, however, are clearly superior to either trial-and-error applications of interventions, which view all interventions as more or less equivalent, or to one-true-light prescriptions, in which one's favored approach is applied to all types and intensities of undesirable behavior. Thus, beginning steps though they may be, certain rudimentary prescriptive guidelines are available to help the teacher determine which procedure to use with which youngster. Because research support is as yet only modest, the reader should view these as suggestive.

1. For youngsters who are only mildly disruptive—those who only occasionally display inappropriate behaviors—extinction will often prove to be the necessary and sufficient intervention.
2. For youngsters who are mildly to moderately disruptive—those who engage in appropriate behavior more than half of the time—procedures for the presentation of positive reinforcement of appropriate behaviors alone will often prove to be the necessary and sufficient intervention.
3. For youngsters who are moderately to severely disruptive—those who engage in appropriate behaviors less than half the time—combined procedures for both the presentation of positive reinforcement of appropriate behaviors and for the removal of positive reinforcement of inappropriate behaviors will often prove to be the necessary and sufficient intervention.

It is the third, moderate-to-severe level of disruptiveness that is most germane to this book. Drawing upon relevant empirical research, Walker (1979) has proposed the following prescriptive hierarchy of interventions of increasing potency for such particularly disruptive, acting-out, or aggressive youngsters. Note that each intervention combines means for both the presentation and removal of positive reinforcement.

1. Teacher praise for appropriate behavior and brief time out for inappropriate behavior (Wasik, Senn, Welch, & Cooper, 1968).
2. Teacher praise and token reinforcement for appropriate behavior and time-out for inappropriate behavior (Walker, Mattson, & Buckley, 1971).
3. Teacher praise for appropriate behavior and response cost for inappropriate behavior (Walker et al., 1976).
4. Teacher praise and positive nonsocial reinforcement for appropriate behavior and response cost for inappropriate behavior (Walker, Street, Garrett, & Crossen, 1977).

Beyond these recommendations, we have three prescriptions to offer. The first are our earlier *semi*prescriptions regarding the optimal use of extinction (p. 90), time-out (p. 93), and response cost (p. 97). The second is the view, also sketched earlier, that modeling, behavioral rehearsal, and similar instructional measures are prescriptively most useful in teaching new behaviors; shaping is especially useful when the person is capable of approximations to appropriate behavior, but no more; and presentations of positive reinforcement fit best when appropriate behaviors have been learned, but for one reason or another are not being performed. Finally, current knowledge allows us to prescribe employment of the least restrictive, least costly, and simplest to implement procedures that seem to hold a reasonable possibility of effective outcome.

TRANSFER AND MAINTENANCE

As we stated at the outset of this chapter, and have reiterated throughout, substantial research evidence exists indicating that singly, and especially in combination, these behavior modification procedures yield high rates of effective behavior change. But questions about transfer and maintenance must be answered less optimistically. Youngsters may indeed change in constructive directions in the classroom in which the given behavior modification procedures were used, but the likelihood that the changes will generalize to other settings (i.e., transfer) or persist over time (i.e., maintenance) is considerably smaller. This frequent failure of gains to either generalize or endure is far from unique to behavioral interventions but, as far as we can discern, applies to almost all educational, psychoeducational, psychological, and psychotherapeutic approaches. For example, in a review of 192 outcome studies that examined the effectiveness of diverse psychotherapies, we commented:

> Though the number of studies . . . reporting positive therapeutic outcomes at the termination of treatment is high (8.55), only 14% of the studies conducted report maintenance or transfer of therapeutic gains. The total sample of studies, furthermore, was selected on criteria reflecting high levels of methodological soundness, thus adding further to the tenability of the conclusion that transfer is a relatively uncommon psychotherapeutic outcome. . . . Keeley, Shemberg, and Carbonell (1976) examined an essentially different series of therapy outcome studies and came to the same conclusion as we have. They focused on the 146 investigations of operant interventions reported in a series of behaviorally oriented journals during 1972–1973. Even moderately long-term concern with transfer was rare. They comment: . . . Only 8 of the 146 studies analyzed present hard data collected at least 6 months past termination, and short term generalization data are conspicuously absent. (Goldstein, Lopez, & Greenleaf, 1979, p. 4)

Successful transfer and maintenance of intervention effects are relatively rare, probably for two reasons. The first is that, as a massive amount of evidence demonstrates, behavior tends to be specific to a situation. That is, behavior tends to be a substantial function of the stimuli and contingencies of the environment in which it occurs. Change the environment and there is an excellent chance behavior will change accordingly. Thus, interventions, including behavior modification interventions, tend to be effective when they are applied but not later (a nonmaintenance effect), and where they are applied but not elsewhere (a nontransfer effect).

The effects of situational specificity of behavior on transfer and maintenance are not immutable however. There is a technology of transfer and maintenance enhancement, a series of tested techniques that may be incorporated into intervention efforts and have been shown to enhance both the generalization and persistence of intervention effects. Our typical failure in most past intervention efforts to draw upon this technology markedly contributes to nontransfer and nonmaintenance. Now that we can do so, however, we can and should substantially increase our success in that regard.

Transfer-Enhancing Procedures

Programmed Generalization

Transfer may be enhanced most directly by efforts that take the intervention which was effective in one setting (e.g., the classroom) and implement it in one or more different settings where the inappropriate behavior also occurs (e.g., the cafeteria, school playground, home). Such an attempt, of course, requires not only additional teacher effort, but possibly the involvement of other teachers, teacher aides, peers, and/or the youngster's parents as additional intervenors.

Using Identical Elements

A youngster will often discriminate between the setting in which the intervention is applied and another in which it is not, because the two settings are markedly dissimilar. He or she may display appropriate behaviors in the former, but not in the latter; transfer in this context will be enhanced only to the degree that the two settings can be made similar. If the intervention cannot be applied in the cafeteria (programmed generalization), temporarily create a cafeteria-like corner in your classroom where you apply your interventions to the young-ster along with the peers with whom he or she associates in the cafeter-ia. More generally, the greater the number of between-settings identical elements you can mobilize, the greater the likely transfer.

Overlearning

Transfer is facilitated the more the youngster has practiced correct or effective use of appropriate behaviors. Behavior modifiers sometimes make the error of using their interventions until a youngster responds correctly, and then they go on to work on other behaviors. Research on overlearning, or overpractice, shows that transfer will be aided if, once a youngster responds in an appropriate manner, he or she is en-couraged to practice the same response several more times. In a sense, we are urging here a strategy of "practice of perfect" to replace the more common "practice makes perfect."

Variety Learning

Transfer is enhanced not only by considerable practice of behaviors, but also when the intervention is mediated by several intervenors and in a variety of settings. Consistent with our earlier observation about inappropriate discriminations, transfer sometimes fails to occur because aspects of the intervention were defined too narrowly. If one intervenor applies a procedure in one setting, the youngster may learn to use ap-propriate behaviors only in that setting and only in response to that intervenor. Transfer, therefore, will be enhanced by using several in-tervenors who apply the intervention across several settings.

Teaching General Principles

Although our emphasis throughout this chapter has been on the modification of specific behaviors, and not just on communicating more abstract guidelines or behavior-change principles, there are youngsters for whom transfer will be promoted by teaching them general rules of conduct. General rules will help more conceptually abstract youngsters decide when and how to use specific behaviors when they find themselves in settings or situations that depart somewhat from the original learning environment.

Maintenance-Enhancing Procedures

Using Intermittent Reinforcement

A well-established principle of behavior modification is that behaviors reinforced intermittently are much more resistant to extinction than are behaviors reinforced continuously. To maintain newly learned appropriate behaviors, then, the strategy should be: (1) to use rich, continuous levels of reinforcement initially to establish the behavior in the youngster's repertoire; (2) to shift as soon as possible to reinforcing the behavior every second or third time it occurs; and (3) to make a subsequent gradual shift to providing reinforcement for the behavior on only an occasional, highly intermittent basis.

Teaching Reinforceable Behaviors

The maintenance of behavior change will be enhanced if teacher decisions about which appropriate behaviors to be developed in the classroom reflect awareness of which appropriate behaviors are likely to be reinforced in other settings. Emphasize those appropriate behaviors that are likely to be relevant to and rewarded elsewhere in the school setting as well as at home, play, or other out-of-school contexts.

Creating New Reinforcements

Maintenance may be facilitated by exposing the youngster to potential reinforcers not chosen by him or her earlier, but nevertheless of possible value or attractiveness. This method works, for example, with youngsters who are minimally responsive at first to social reinforcement but who develop responsiveness to praise, approval, and its other manifestations when the presentation of social reinforcement is consistently paired with presentations of material, activity, or token reinforcement.

Reprogramming the Environment

Combining several of the features of the transfer-enhancing techniques of programmed generalization and variety learning, reprogramming the environment consists of having the main figures in the youngster's out-of-class environment collaborate in implementing the intervention in as many settings as possible. Other teachers, the youngster's parents, peers, and others may all profitably join in this maintenance-enhancing effort.

Using Self-Reinforcement

A youngster will often use a newly learned appropriate behavior correctly in an out-of-class setting and not be reinforced for the effort. A different teacher may ignore the behavior; peers may prefer the antisocial to the prosocial; parents may feel that the behavior is simply expected and deserves no special recognition. Whatever the sources of potential extinction, appropriate behaviors are more likely to be maintained under these circumstances when the youngster has been taught to give himself or herself what have been termed "self-messages" to the effect that he or she "did a good job" or "handled the situation well" or some similar self-reinforcing message. Developers of this technique have suggested furthermore that following the use of particularly difficult appropriate behaviors, the youngster might well not only say reinforcing things to himself or herself, but may also provide himself or herself with a desired material or activity reinforcer.

Transfer and maintenance enhancement are a crucial component of any behavior modification effort, and thus we strongly urge their inclusion in classroom attempts to deal effectively with aggressive and disruptive youngsters. Further information regarding these transfer- and maintenance-enhancing techniques, as well as others, are provided at length in Goldstein and Kanfer (1979) and Karoly and Steffen (1980).

ETHICAL ISSUES

Earlier we alluded to a series of objections that have been raised, on ethical grounds, to the utilization of behavior modification procedures in school settings. At this point, having both described these procedures in detail and underscored their behavior-change potency, we wish to readdress these ethical concerns in greater depth. The substantial, often dramatic effectiveness of behavior modification procedures by no means inexorably dictates that such procedures be used. There are criteria of acceptability which transcend effectiveness, criteria which — in addition to effectiveness — must unequivocally be met prior to the employment of any behavioral or nonbehavioral procedure. Let us see whether behavior modification procedures meet such criteria.

Manipulation

Webster's Encyclopedic Dictionary (1973) defines manipulation as "the act of operating upon skillfully, for the purpose of giving a false appear-ance to" (p. 515). Unfortunately, what we perceive to be the all-too-frequent naive use of behavior modification has provided evidence for this negative view of behavioral technology as the clever (some would say Machiavellian) but not very thorough or long-lasting manipulation of surface behavior. In fact, we would agree that when behavior modifi-cation is used, as it sometimes is, by uninformed adults in a cursory and unthoughtful way to control the behavior of other adults or of chil-dren, then Webster's definition may indeed apply. There is, however, another perspective on manipulation. With a small but significant change in its dictionary definition, we would grant that behavior modifi-cation is indeed manipulative. Were one to replace "false" in this defi-nition with "changed," we would clearly label behavior modification as manipulation. Furthermore, in this altered definition, the term manipulation is in our view very far from a term of disapproval. In our sense of the term, all educational, psychological, and psychoeduca-tional interventions are and should be manipulative — the behavioral, the psychodynamic, the humanistic, and all others. Where approaches differ is in how effective their efforts are, and how open intervenors are — both to others and especially to themselves — to the notion that they are indeed "operating upon skillfully, for the purpose of giving a changed appearance to." Referring to therapeutic applications of be-havior modification, O'Leary and Wilson (1975) have reflected this view-point well in their observation:

> Behavior modification is often indicted for supposedly denying individual freedom and for being a mechanistic, manipulative, and impersonal ap-proach which deliberately sets out to control behavior. On the other hand, purportedly more humanistic forms of therapy are applauded because they claim to promote individual "growth" or "self-actualization" without imposing any external control. What such a comparison overlooks is the now widely accepted truism that all forms of therapy involve control or social influence. Truax (1966), for example, has shown how even Carl Rogers' "nondirective" therapy results in the therapist unwittingly rein-

forcing particular types of client verbalizations which the therapist believes to be therapeutic. The issue is not whether clients' behavior should or should not be controlled; it unquestionably is. The important question then becomes whether the therapist is aware of this control and the behaviors it is used to develop. (pp. 28–29)

Precisely the same point may be made about the everyday behavior of the typical classroom teacher. By presenting or withholding approval, smiling, staring, touching, scolding, praising, giving permission to engage in pleasurable activities, denying opportunity for such activities, and in literally dozens of other ways, the teacher functions as a highly active, highly influential, highly manipulative (in our revised definitional sense) modifier of his or her students' behavior. Manipulation is present. Its effective and efficient utilization often are not. We hope this presentation of behavior modification procedures will serve as a small contribution to enhancing the effectiveness of their utilization.

Freedom of Choice

The technology of behavior modification has been criticized by some for resulting in a diminution of the target person's freedom of choice. Other people (the intervenor), it is held, act upon the person and, by the effective use of behavior modification procedures, choose for that person the behaviors he or she comes to utilize. In our view, this is the least cogent argument against the ethics of behavior modification. In fact, on the contrary, enhanced, not diminished, freedom of choice is the net consequence of behavioral interventions for target youngsters. Intervenors only choose the procedures for reaching goal behaviors, that is, the "how" of behavior modification. The goals themselves, or the "what" of this intervention, as well as the "why" and "when" are at least in some instances selected not only by the teacher, the teacher's school, and community at large but, when done properly, by the youngster himself or herself. Participation by the target youngster in goal-behavior selection is not always possible and is sometimes inappropriate. But in a great many interventions which behaviors are to be pinpointed for modification will be a decision to which the youngster contributes substantially.

There is a second, equally significant way in which successful behavior modification produces enhanced freedom of choice. It does so by enlarging the target individual's behavioral repertoire. Prior to the successful application of, let us say, positive reinforcement for negotiating differences with a fellow student and time out for physically brawling with peers, a youngster may well be essentially without choice when faced with a dispute. That is, his or her prepotent response — to lash out, punch, fight — may be his or her only potential response.

Negotiation of disputes, calling upon others, withdrawal, or other possible and less aggressive responses may never have been used by the youngster, or may have been used exceedingly rarely, and hence for all practical purposes may not be alternatives he or she might call upon by choice. In essence, not knowing alternatives, the youngster has no choice. He or she *must* fight. When the behavioral intervention succeeds in increasing the likelihood of negotiation as a response by arming the youngster with a new alternative, the youngster is correspondingly armed with the ability to choose. Now he or she may fight or negotiate as he or she chooses, and as he or she perceives the potential rewards and punishments of the two (or more) alternatives. The decision to use reinforcement and time-out was largely the teacher's; the decision to reward negotiation behavior was, we hope, jointly the teacher's and the youngster's. But the decision to actually negotiate a dispute with a peer is and should be wholly the youngster's. Thus, the heart of our view is that by means of collaborating when possible in decisions about target behaviors to be modified, and by unilaterally deciding when to use newly learned (and heretofore unavailable, thus unchoosable) appropriate behaviors, behavior modification is indeed a choice-enhancing technology.

Bribery

The accusation that those behavior modification procedures that present reinforcement for appropriate behaviors are equivalent to the use of bribery also seems erroneous to us. Bribery is defined as a prize, gift, or other favor bestowed or promised to pervert the judgment or corrupt the conduct of a person (Webster, 1973). In behavior modification, reinforcement is used neither to pervert nor corrupt but, instead, to reward and broaden the person's repertoire of personally and socially useful behaviors. A reward for the prosocial differs greatly in an ethical sense from one presented for the antisocial.

Yet the objection is still raised that youngsters should not need an external reward for doing what society expects them to do. Instead, negotiating disputes, paying attention, remaining in one's seat, speaking conversationally, not cursing, not fighting, and other desirable classroom behaviors should be intrinsically rewarding. This view, we feel, is both hypocritical and factually incorrect. It is hypocritical because reward is presented for appropriate behavior at all other levels of society—often including teachers for their appropriate teaching behaviors, and to these same youngsters by these same teachers (in albeit unsystematic form) every teaching day. We also think it is factually incorrect that "youngster's should not need an external reward for doing what society expects them to do," because, simply put, some literally don't know what society expects. This generalization applies to many types of youngsters with special needs, and most certainly includes the chronically aggressive, disruptive, acting-out youngster of special concern to us here.

Whose Needs Are Served?

A further ethical concern pertains to decisions about whose needs will take precedence when choices must be made about whether to employ behavior modification procedures in a given classroom, and about how to use them when they are employed. Among the earliest applied uses of behavior modification were attempts to employ it in mental hospitals to alter the behavior of long-term, adult psychiatric patients. Literally hundreds of research papers attest to the success of this effort. But which behaviors were altered? How was success defined? In far too large a percentage of these investigations, the "appropriate" behaviors successfully developed were patient behaviors whose occurrence met the needs of the staff (the intervenors) at least as much and often more than the patient's. "Good patient" behaviors were rewarded, that is, those behaviors that included patient compliance, passivity, and dependency, and led to an orderly and predictable ward, one relatively comfortable and manageable for the staff. Such a regime, which has come to be appropriately known as a "colonization effect" for its robotizing influence upon patients, ill prepared such patients for the demands of community living when the deinstitutionalization movement led to 400,000 of them (between 1965 and 1980) being discharged from America's public mental hospitals.

This apparent digression into the adult mental health realm is in fact relevant to our question, "Whose needs will be served?" Will it be the school's at large? The teacher's? The youngster's? Although it would be naive to argue that schools have not made use of behavior modification as a powerful tool to teach "good student" behaviors (analogous to "good patient" behaviors), it would be equally foolish, in our view, to throw out the technology because some schools and teachers have misused it. If our goal is to be truly helpful to youngsters and to enhance the educational and emotional potential of our students, not just to maintain an orderly and manageable classroom, we submit that

teachers should and will make the decision to employ appropriate behavior modification procedures with aggressive and other special-needs
youngsters, and to apply them toward the development of appropriate behaviors that will contribute not only to a calm classroom climate,
but will also serve the youngster well both within school and elsewhere.

RESPONSIVENESS TO RESEARCH

Behavior modification has suffered from bad press and bad public relations. Behavior modification — the specific procedures described in
this chapter — has been both confused with Machiavellian fictional accounts of its substance (e.g., *A Clockwork Orange*) and identified with other
existing procedures that also seek to change behavior but by means
having nothing whatsoever in common with behavior modification (e.g.,
psychosurgery, sterilization). This negative public image is all the more
surprising when one recognizes the vast and almost unique level of empirical support that exists attesting to the real world effectiveness of
this approach. No other existing means for altering, influencing, or
modifying human behavior in appropriate directions rests on a com-
parably broad and deep empirical foundation. We believe that one of
our highest ethical responsibilities is to be responsive to objective evidence, to offer our students the benefits of what research has repeatedly demonstrated to be effective, to try to overcome our own biases,
and to act in the welfare of others in ways that are most clearly indicated by cumulative scientific evidence. Meeting this ethical responsibility will often mean modifying teacher behavior, and that will be reflected
in greater utilization of behavior modification programs based on the
thoughtful application of appropriate principles to the diverse
manifestations of school violence. Finally, we must be careful that we
do not oversell this approach, however empirically based or utilitarian it appears to be. Although we have demonstrated that behavior
modification programs are often able to document their success in
teaching appropriate behaviors to children and adults, much empirical work remains to be done. It is our hope that the creative researcher and thoughtful teacher will join together in responding to this
challenge.

NOTE

1. Most of the Mediation-Reinforcer Incomplete Blank items help specify
not only the nature of the events the youngster perceives as positive reinforcers, but also who are the mediators of such reinforcers — highly important in-

formation in carrying out a contingency management effort. Going to a ball game may be a powerful reinforcer if accompanied by peers, a weak one if taken there by one's teacher or mother. Praise from a respected teacher may be a potent reinforcing event, whereas the same praise delivered by a peer considered by the youngster as ignorant with regard to the behavior involved may be totally lacking in potency.

Psychodynamic and Humanistic Interventions

In their review of research on crime in schools, McPartland and McDill (1977) identified five major themes in theories of youth crime:

1. The theme of *restricted opportunity* emphasizes the barriers many young people must hurdle to achieve the good jobs, material possessions, and status that symbolize the American dream. In this view, criminal acts are representative of youngsters' frustration directed at the system that holds them back. Schools are easily identifiable targets.

2. The theme of *subcultural differences in values and attitudes* posits that, for whatever reason, subcultures exist in which middle-class values and aspirations are rejected and crime and violence are a fact of life. In neighborhoods and communities in which the deviant subculture takes hold, residents are continually exposed to violent behaviors and the supports needed to combat such actions are minimal.

3. The third theme, *prolonged adolescent dependence,* is based on the contradictory experience of most teenagers in America today. Even though many adolescents have the ability to take on substantial adult responsibilities, society seems to provide little place for their contributions. The frustrations engendered by adolescents as the result of this state of affairs may often find an outlet in delinquent behaviors designed to demonstrate independence.

4. The fourth theme states that *seriously damaged personalities,* more than environmental and societal conditions, are the basis for the most serious criminal behaviors among youth. Delinquency, in this view, is

the expression of the individual's inability to control his or her own aggressive and antisocial impulses. Youngsters who commit violent criminal acts are held to be seriously emotionally disturbed.

5. According to the theme of *labeling and stereotyping*, a youngster may come to view himself or herself as criminal or delinquent or "bad" because others in authority continually communicate that image to him or her. Such a process may be viewed as an example of a self-fulfilling prophecy in which the imposition of a label sets in motion a chain of events that validates the label or stereotype.

Although McPartland and McDill note that the first three themes just listed (restricted opportunity, subcultural differences, and prolonged adolescent dependence) are primarily sociological in nature, and the last two themes (seriously damaged personalities, and labeling and stereotyping) more psychologically based, each of the five themes may be viewed in relation to a psychodynamic perspective. Such a viewpoint seeks to understand human nature through analysis of the internal processes and forces which are assumed to be the basis for behavior.

In this view, deviant behavior is a symptom of unresolved (and usually unconscious) underlying disturbances and often occurs when the individual's control system is unable to regulate his or her impulses. Thus, the youngster who commits a violent or criminal act may have failed to successfully work through the intrapsychic conflicts that he or she faced in the process of psychological and physical development.

Consequently, whether causation is restricted opportunity that heightens frustration and aggressive impulses, or a deviant subculture that weakens internal controls, or prolonged adolescent dependence that places extra strains on an already overloaded developmental period, a psychodynamic position can be useful in understanding motivations and in developing interventions. Such a perspective can be equally helpful in our efforts to understand seriously damaged personalities and the effects of labeling and stereotyping on youngsters' self-concepts.

In this chapter, we examine the psychodynamic point of view as originally conceptualized by Freud and others as it bears upon student aggression. In addition, we focus on one of the major outgrowths of psychodynamic theory: humanistic psychology. Although there is much to be discussed regarding the application of psychodynamic principles to the problems of aggressive and violent behavior in schools, the professional literature does not provide many examples of controlled and data-based studies that might offer valid and reliable evidence of the effectiveness of psychodynamic techniques. Nevertheless, as we shall see, the psychodynamic approach has had an enormous impact on clinical and educational efforts to serve troubled youngsters.

THE PSYCHODYNAMIC POSITION

According to Chess and Hassibi (1978):

> The central concepts of psychoanalytic theory can be described as follows: all behavior, thoughts, feelings, acts, dreams, and fantasies—whether normal or pathological, rational or accidental—are motivated and meaningful, even though the motivation may be obscure and the meaning not easily discerned. The ultimate motivating forces in all behavioral phenomena are the instinctual drives. Because the immediate and direct gratification of these drives is incompatible with the social existence of man, the individual must develop indirect means and compromises to adapt to external reality and find acceptable ways of gratification. Conflict is therefore the inevitable component of the intrapsychic life of the individual.
>
> The most important instinctual drive in psychoanalytic theory is sexuality (libido). Aggression is postulated as another basic instinct.... Instinctual drives are viewed as possessing energy. Although nonquantifiable, this energy is like an electrical charge that propels every aspect of behavior. (p. 46)

We can see in the preceding quotation that the core of the psychodynamic position is the continual conflict between inner impulses and the individual's efforts to control, or at least ensure, the socially acceptable gratification of his or her instinctual drives. As each infant grows and develops, reality demands increase and immediate gratification becomes more difficult to attain. A conscious self begins to develop to control the infant's unconscious wishes and demands.

In order to fully understand psychodynamic thought, then, one must be aware of the three major personality systems: the *id, ego,* and *superego*—three hypothetical constructs that form the basis of psychological development in this view. The id represents instinctual energy (it is the only system present at birth) and its power is used in the service of the "pleasure principle" (the constant effort to achieve gratification and to avoid pain). The superego represents societal values and often conflicts directly with the id. The ego serves as the mediating system, working through the conflicts between the id and superego by the use of logic and rationality (the "reality principle"), in an effort to control or neutralize the impulses of the id.

When the three systems work together productively, the person is able to meet his or her needs without trespassing on others' rights or society's rules, and he or she is said to be well-adjusted. When the systems are in conflict—if, for example, the id's impulses are too strong to control—then the person is said to be maladjusted and deviant behavior may result.

It is also necessary to understand the role of anxiety in the psychodynamic position. When instinctual drives, in the effort to find immediate gratification, threaten to overwhelm the ego, the arousal of anxiety is the likely result. When this occurs, the ego must redouble its control efforts, using one or more of the defense mechanisms (repression, regression, rationalization, sublimation, etc.) to reassert control over the id. When the efforts of the ego fail and the impulses of the id are allowed to proceed unchecked, personality disorganization, deviant behavior, and other symptoms of emotional disturbance frequently appear.

Reinert (1976) summarizes it this way:

> From a psychodynamic point of view the child in conflict has not negotiated, at a successful level, the various intrapsychic and external conflicts that he faced in the process of psychological and/or physiological maturity. (p. 93)

In addition to the three major personality systems, psychoanalytic thought is also based on a sequence of five psychosexual developmental stages. Beginning from birth, the stages are: *oral, anal, phallic, latency,* and *genital.* Each child passes relatively systematically through the developmental stages, though some overlapping of stages does occur. Though it is not uncommon for problems to occur even in the development of typical children, disturbed youngsters often fail to resolve the dilemmas presented by one or another of the psychosexual stages.

From a psychodynamic perspective, the first three stages are critical, because by the time the youngster has completed the phallic stage the basic personality components have been established. If problems have been resolved successfully in those early years, later difficulties are less likely. Problem behaviors might develop because a child invests too much psychic energy in one stage and has insufficient resources to meet the next, or a youngster has difficulty at later stages and may regress to behavior characteristics of earlier times.

In their classic follow-up study of juvenile delinquents, Glueck and Glueck (1940) noted that many of the offenders whom they studied could be viewed as fixated at earlier levels of development:

> In fact, from many angles the conduct of not a few offenders, when passed in review over the years, may be regarded as infantile: witness their impulsiveness, their lack of playfulness, their failure to postpone immediate desires for more distant ones, their incapacity or unwillingness to profit by numerous experiences of punishment or correction, the excessive attachment of many of them to their mothers, their inability to assume marital, family, and other responsibilities appropriate to their chronological age. (p. 268)

In addition to Freud's psychosexual stages just described, Erikson (1950) developed a sequence of eight psychosocial stages based on the developing individual's changing social relationships. In Erikson's view, psychological health and pathology are determined as much by the individual's relation to society as they are by his or her inner conflicts. Again, in order from birth, those stages are: *basic trust versus mistrust, autonomy versus shame and doubt, initiative versus guilt, industry versus inferiority, identity versus identity diffusion, intimacy versus isolation, generativity versus stagnation, and ego integration versus despair.* Because progress through the psychosocial developmental stages is so individualized, dependent as it is on unconscious internal impulses and the idiosyncratic events of one's external environments, each person develops a unique personal history that is critical to an understanding of behavior.

According to Morse, Smith, and Acker (1977), the assumptions made by the psychodynamic viewpoint — that unconscious internal impulses and forces motivate human behavior, that personality is dynamic and develops in terms of psychosexual and psychosocial stages, and that each person develops a unique psychological history — have important implications for work with children who commit deviant acts:

> These assumptions have important implications for educators. First, we expect that children of the same chronological age will be at different developmental levels, and that they may regress at times to earlier stages. Second, children have different degrees of knowledge and control over their internal motivating forces. Third, behaviors which appear to be abnormal may actually be normal for a child at a particular developmental stage. Fourth, a child's behavior in any setting is indicative of strong underlying needs and impulses. (pp. 12–13)

One basic premise of the psychodynamic model is that disturbed behavior is determined by psychological processes. Psychopathology is determined by the way in which the individual's psychological makeup — thoughts, feelings, perceptions, needs, and so on — responds to the events of everyday life. Though everyone brings inherited potentialities to life situations, it is the specific manner in which those genetic or biological factors interact with particular aspects of the individual's own life that results in the development of maladaptive or disturbed behavior.

Long (1966) has developed a framework for understanding the interaction between biological potential and environmental influences previously described. According to Long's cycle, each child's innate inherited potential is soon subjected to the stresses and strains of the youngster's environment, with anxiety the likely result. The youngster's efforts to ward off the anxiety by employing one or another of the defense mechanisms usually results in increased conflicts, especially in school settings. Consequently, that conflict produces more anxiety and the cycle is repeated continuously.

In summary, the following characteristics are important aspects of the psychodynamic viewpoint:

1. All behavior—thoughts, feelings, acts, dreams, and so on—is meaningful though the meaning is not always clear to the person or to an observer. The meaning must be understood in order to develop effective behavior—change interventions.

2. All children have some basic needs that must be met in order to develop healthy personalities. These include the need for food and shelter, love, security, belonging, success, and so on.

3. The quality of the emotional relationship a child has with his or her family and other significant people in his or her life is of crucial significance.

4. Each child goes through several stages of emotional growth. Traumatic experiences and deprivations may interfere with this growth and result in lasting personality disturbances.

5. Anxiety over unmet needs and inner conflicts is an important determinant in behavior disorders. The individual's ability to cope with anxiety is critical.

6. Behaviors that reflect a state of emotional disturbance are caused primarily by internal psychic pathology—conflicts between impulses and controls.

7. Both biological forces and early environmental influences contribute to the pathological condition.

PSYCHODYNAMIC INTERVENTIONS

Although it is difficult to find a body of work in the professional literature in which psychodynamic formulations are used as the basis of intervention efforts aimed at reducing school violence, the psychodynamic viewpoint, nonetheless, has had an impact on efforts to control aggressive behavior in schools. When youngsters commit violent or aggressive acts in school in sufficient numbers or in sufficient intensity to require intervention by school authorities, it is likely that those youngsters will be viewed as emotionally disturbed. When we examine the history of interventions with youngsters labeled emotionally disturbed, it is easy to see the wide-ranging impact of the psychodynamic point of view.

For many years, at the beginning of the short history of educating disturbed children, the psychodynamic model represented the only point of view in the field. Juul (1977) noted that the early, exclusive use of the model created the following lasting impact:

1. With its revelations of the rich and complex inner life of children, it has created in parents and teachers a new sensitivity to children's feelings and needs.

2. The discoveries of the devastating effects that emotional deprivation in early childhood has on personality development led to major reforms in child care institutions and agencies.

3. Teachers have become conscious about their importance to their pupils as models and as objects of identification. They also realize that through their relations with their children they can alleviate many emotional problems and create security and confidence. (pp. 13–14)

Psychodynamic theory has thus had a very significant influence on work with troubled children. Some specific applications include: *milieu therapy; life space interviewing; play therapy; art, music, and dance therapy; classrooms in psychiatric clinics;* and many more. According to Newcomer (1980), the psychodynamic model has emphasized the premise that personality characteristics are determined by early childhood events. For disturbed youngsters, this implies that emotional distress is caused in early family relationships and that school problems are simply repeat manifestations of those early disturbances. As a result, psychodynamic thinking has focused considerably on child- and family-intervention strategies—not school interventions.

Newcomer (1980) also notes that psychodynamic models are based on the notion "that abnormal behaviors are symptoms of unconscious conflict" (p. 38). Consequently, educators must realize that troubled children are frequently not conscious of the rationale or motivation for their inappropriate behavior, nor are they able to consciously control that behavior. From this view, then, an additional implication is that treatment of symptoms (overt behavior) may simply result in the substitution of other more problematic symptoms and should thus be avoided. Instead, youngsters should be encouraged to express their feelings, and educators should be trained to provide environments that do not repress youngsters' symptomatology and their opportunities to express the underlying conflicts.

Newcomer (1980) summarizes the positive contributions of the psychodynamic model as follows:

1. Children do not always consciously plan and cannot always consciously control disruptive behaviors, therefore when they misbehave they should not be treated punitively;

2. Hostility directed to the teacher should not be viewed as a personal insult since it might stem from a variety of motivations and does not necessarily mean that the child dislikes the teacher;
3. Children respond to internal conflicts, therefore, inconsistencies in behavior should be expected. (p. 38)

As we have seen, the psychodynamic viewpoint treats deviant behavior as the product of conflict between a child's impulse system and his or her control system. When impulses overwhelm controls, the child's behavior may be aggressive and unpredictable. When the control system is overdeveloped and impulses (even positive ones) are constantly quashed, the child may be inhibited and withdrawn. Consequently, depending on the nature of the youngster's difficulty, interventions may attempt either to help the child learn to express positive impulses appropriately and/or to develop appropriate and effective controls.

According to Morse et al. (1977), the goals of psychodynamic interventions with troubled children may be internal, behavioral, or environmental. Internal goals focus on changes in the youngster's feelings about himself or herself and others. Behavioral goals may center on efforts to help children control negative impulses in order to express feelings in socially acceptable ways. Environmental goals include attempts to provide children with surroundings that offer the emotional supports needed for positive growth and development.

In all cases, psychodynamic interventions assume that:

1. The youngster is usually not consciously aware of the source of his or her problem.
2. Changing surface behavior is less important than dealing with underlying conflicts.
3. Change requires the development of insight into past and present conflicts and the development of new and more productive patterns of behavior.
4. Treatment for pathological behaviors is typically long and difficult.

To a great extent, the application of psychodynamic principles to the remediation of aggressive behavior in school-age children and youth may be traced to the work of Fritz Redl and his colleagues. Redl's work with delinquent youngsters in the 1940s and 1950s served as the impetus for the creation of a variety of techniques for the control of aggressive behavior. He has also reaffirmed the psychodynamic emphasis on understanding underlying motivations as a necessary beginning to the planning of interventions (Redl, 1969). Such an emphasis can be seen clearly in Redl's discussion of the differences between three kinds of aggression that youngsters may display in school:

> First, a teenager gets hopping mad at his old man, but he doesn't dare let off steam until he gets to school. Now, the teacher didn't produce the aggression, but he's there and he's got to handle it.
>
> Second, is the discharge from within. Some youngsters sit there daydreaming, and all of a sudden during a wild fantasy, he thinks of something that upsets him and he conks his neighbors on the head. None of them have done anything to him, and the teacher hasn't either. Something just burst out from within. (If youngsters are seriously disturbed, most of the aggression comes from way within, and neither they nor anyone else knows why.)
>
> Third, the aggression is engendered right there in the classroom. It may be triggered either by what the teacher does that's right but that doesn't happen to fit the kid, or by God knows what—the kid's reaction to the group or to other kids, or to something that maybe the teacher wouldn't have done if he had stopped to think. But anyway, it's reactive to something in the environment at the moment.
>
> Now, if I were a classroom teacher, I would like to know how much of which of those three packages is exploding before me, because it makes a difference in terms of long-range planning. It also makes some difference in terms of what to do at the moment. . . . The way Joe or Jane expresses aggression, while not the end of what we're looking for, certainly should be the starting point. Unless you know what lies behind their behavior, you will have trouble knowing how to handle it. (pp. 30–31)

Redl's psychodynamic view of aggressive behavior is based on the premise that aggressive youngsters have failed to develop appropriate ego skills. As a result of such disturbances in their control systems, aggressive youngsters, in Redl's view, tend to make more than their share of faulty decisions. Frequently, such children are overwhelmed by inner impulses and find themselves unable to suppress or divert the inappropriate expression of feelings. The actions that result are often antisocial and unacceptable and have the net effect of causing further problems for the youngster in question. In turn, the youngster's likely reaction to these predicaments is even more inappropriate behavior, because his or her control system is simply unable to deal effectively with the anxiety aroused by the worsening conflict.

Interventions for such youngsters, according to Redl, fall into two major categories: assisting youngsters in the control of their aggressive impulses (manipulations of surface behavior) and helping youngsters develop better understanding of their own motivations and the options available to them for more appropriate expressions of feelings (clinical exploitation of life events). We discuss each of these intervention categories in turn, but it is important first to point out that both kinds of interventions are based on two essential principles:

1. *Interpersonal relationships are essential to positive psychological growth and development.* Youngsters with deficient ego skills are particularly unlikely to have developed rewarding relationships, and adults who intend to intervene effectively with such children should focus on the development of a relationship right from the start. This effort is essential because the adult must often "lend" his or her own ego skills to the youngster and provide the controls which the youngster has yet to develop. In addition, the development of a positive adult–child relationship can make the adult's messages more "receivable" by the youngster (If I can see that you care about me, maybe it's worth considering what you have to say or modeling some of your actions.)

2. *Program planning is critical in efforts with troubled youngsters.* What kinds of activities to plan, and for what particular purposes, and for which children, are questions adults must continually ask themselves. Redl and others who espouse a psychodynamic viewpoint are most concerned with the mental hygiene goals of programming—that is, the ability of planned activities to help youngsters drain off excessive impulsive energy, avoid frustration, reduce the threat of new situations, accept gradually increasing levels of organization, and so on. Thus, programs must be planned for the dual purpose of supporting egos, deficient though they may be, while at the same time working to increase a wide range of important ego skills and strengths.

We turn now to a more extensive discussion of Redl's techniques for assisting youngsters in the control of their aggressive impulses.

ANTISEPTIC MANIPULATIONS OF SURFACE BEHAVIOR

Redl and Wineman (1957) note that whereas clinicians have often been concerned with long-term change of strongly rooted problems through the slow dissolution of causal chains, educators and others who spend their days with aggressive children are more concerned with learning how to stop youngsters' inappropriate behavior immediately. Redl and Wineman further note three major reasons for the amalgamation of clinical and educational practices:

1. Regardless of the long-term therapeutic goal, reality demands interference into a variety of child behaviors. Obviously, youngsters about to hurt themselves or others, regardless of the underlying motivation impelling them to do so, must be stopped.

2. Behaviors that call for immediate intervention also require antiseptic manipulation; in addition to being effective, the techniques utilized must not do harm to the overall clinical goals.

3. Planned interference can be a clinical tool itself, not just an unavoidable compromise of valid therapeutic technique. Total permissiveness is not the wisest clinical policy for such youngsters and the right kind of intervention applied at the proper place and time may be just what is needed.

On the basis of the rationale just outlined, Redl and Wineman described seventeen ways in which inappropriate surface behaviors can be antiseptically manipulated, which are outlined below.

Planned Ignoring

Because much of the children's behavior that may be bothersome to adults is often abandoned by the child when he or she ceases receiving the adult's interest, adults can help decrease the intensity and/or frequency of such behavior by not attending to it, that is, by planned ignoring of the behavior. Interestingly, although this is a principle of behavioral intervention developed in a psychodynamic perspective, note that planned ignoring is also an essential element of the behavioral position described elsewhere in this book (see extinction, p. 90). Redl and Wineman point out that even though it is easy to think of examples of behavior that can profitably be ignored, the deceptively simple skill of knowing which behaviors to ignore is an extremely important asset for those who work with aggressive children.

Signal Interference

A great deal of aggressive behavior may occur because a youngster's control system has not been alerted to rapidly developing provocation in the environment. In such cases, an adult can arrest the behavior by signaling its unacceptability in a friendly and nonthreatening way. The adult's signal reactivates the youngster's control system and the inappropriate behavior is not expressed.

Proximity and Touch Control

Under certain conditions, physical proximity lends support to the youngster's ego and consequently to the maintenance of appropriate behavior even in the face of temptation. This intervention may be viewed as a continuum, with some youngsters who respond to more active expressions of closeness (i.e., touch control) and some who need only minimal evidence of adult nearness (simply the presence of the adult in the general area) in order to control their behavior.

Involvement in Interest Relationship

Youngsters with ego disturbances, according to Redl and Wineman (1957), "seem to need a more constant revival of the vitality of their interest fields by direct adult participation" (p. 410). Adults can divert inappropriate behaviors by demonstrating interest in more socially acceptable uses of a new toy or otherwise showing interest in those things that interest the child.

Hypodermic Affection

Sometimes youngsters need a burst of affection or love to help their egos retain control of their impulses. For example, if a youngster's aggressiveness increases because of the fear that he or she is not liked, a "shot of love" is likely to be a more effective intervention than a more typical adult reaction to the aggressive act itself.

Tension Decontamination Through Humor

Sometimes, despite the intensity of a youngster's ego impairment, he or she can be "kidded out of" performing aggressive or violent acts. Redl and Wineman posit that humor is probably effective because it demonstrates the invulnerability of the adult to the child's destructive impulses; it saves the child from the retaliation and/or guilt that might have followed the inappropriate behavior; it enables the youngster to save face, and so on. Whatever the reason, humor can be an effective way to stop the aggressive behavior and the production of secondary complications (i.e., contagion to other members of the group).

Hurdle Help

Aggressive outbursts may result from the inability of the control system to withstand the impulses generated by certain frustration-producing events. When goal-directed behavior is blocked, torrents of inappropriate behavior may be a troubled child's only available response. In such cases, adults can prevent the occurrence of aggression by timely efforts to help youngsters hurdle the obstacles in their paths. This is a particularly useful intervention in school programs, as the sensitive educator realizes, for example, that a child's inability to complete the first problem in a math test might result in the expression of considerable aggressive behavior.

Interpretation as Interference

Simply stated, this technique involves the use of interpretation to help a youngster understand a particular situation and his or her own contribution to it. Ultimately, of course, the purpose is to stop inappropriate behavior by interpreting it to the child. Redl and Wineman point out that this technique is effective only when there is a possibility that a youngster might act differently if he or she understood the situation differently.

Regrouping

Because problem behavior may stem from the psychological makeup of the group, changing the composition of that group may reduce the incidence of aggressive and violent episodes. This may be done on at least three different levels: *total regrouping* in which a particular youngster is placed in a different setting because of the failure to match him or her to an appropriate group in the first setting; *partial regrouping* that involves a shift in the composition of a group within the setting; and *distributional changes* that simply alter the responsibilities and interactions within a group without necessitating a change in membership.

Restructuring

Sometimes even the most carefully planned programs do not work out as intended. In these cases, even "normal" children are known to respond by acting out and sensitive adults realize the need to restructure the activity. For example if youngsters become restless because they have had to sit still for a prolonged period, a wise teacher or group leader will change to a more active format.

Direct Appeal

Perhaps because youngsters with ego disturbances are often viewed as lacking in inner understanding, there is a tendency to underutilize the technique of direct appeal. Redl and Wineman point out, however, that once relationships between children and adults begin to develop, use of a direct appeal may be more effective than many adults realize. Depending on the youngster and his or her relationship to the adult, appeals might be made on a variety of bases, including personal relationships, physical reality, outsiders' sensitivities, values, the group code, narcissistic pride, personal considerations, and others.

Limitation of Space and Tools

This technique has two levels. First, problem behavior can often be prevented by the strategic limitation of space and tools. For example, it is clearly seductive to leave cash or potentially dangerous implements where youngsters with inadequate control mechanisms have easy access to them, and to the problems that will likely occur when impulses overwhelm controls. Second, when inappropriate behavior occurs as the result of the inappropriate use of space or tools, intervention of this sort (taking the tool away, refusing entrance to the space, etc.) may be necessary.

Antiseptic Bouncing

Under certain circumstances, the removal of a child from the scene of conflict may be the only way to intervene. Redl and Wineman caution that this technique ought to be used in situations of an emergency nature, as well as to prevent emergencies from occurring, and must be done without anger and hostility on the adult's part. For example, antiseptic bouncing may be called for when clear physical dangers exist, when the youngster's very presence stirs up unending contagion to other group members or makes it impossible for the youngster to calm down, or when the issue is so critical that a clear demonstration of limits by the adult is mandated.

Physical Restraint

Some youngsters are prone to violent fits of rage characterized by hitting, kicking, biting, screaming, swearing, lashing out, and so on. This total loss of control may occur spontaneously and it is often difficult for adults to understand the precipitating factors. Redl and Wineman point out that the major concern with such episodes is that the child's loss of control makes it impossible to communicate with his or her ego and renders adults powerless. Whatever relationship may have developed between adult and child vanishes temporarily in the rage of the moment.

At such times, the only useful adult intervention may be physical restraint. This is to be done reasonably but firmly and should not be viewed as in any way related to physical punishment. The adult must use no more force than is absolutely necessary to restrain the youngster's inappropriate behavior. In Redl and Wineman's (1957) words, the attitude to be conveyed refuses to take the child's wild behavior seriously:

> Listen, kid, this is nuts. There is not the slightest reality reason for you to act that way. We like you. There is nothing to fear, but there is also nothing to gain by such behavior. You didn't get us mad by it, for we know you can't help it right now. But we sure hope this will reduce as time goes on. We aren't holding it against you, either. We want only one thing: get it over with, snap back into your more reasonable self, so we can communicate with you again. (p. 454)

Clearly, though Redl and Wineman would not use these words with the youngster in need of restraint, they emphasize the importance of applying physical restraint antiseptically. This is done by demonstrating a valuing of the person and a refusal to acknowledge the wild and aggressive behavior as characteristic of the child's true personality.

Permission and "Authoritative Verbot"

The use of permission falls into three categories: (1) to begin a piece of appropriate behavior that might otherwise have been blocked, (2) to reduce the occurrence of behavior that was meant to irritate or antagonize, or to keep an activity at a manageable level and within tolerable limits, and (3) "authoritative verbot," which is simply a flowery term for the clear, firm, and unequivocal "no" which behavior sometimes mandates but adults may be hesitant to express. Again, this must be expressed antiseptically, without adult anger or anxiety, and in a friendly—not challenging—tone.

Promises and Rewards

From a psychodynamic point of view, the pleasure principle indicates that youngsters, even those with severe ego disturbances, will be inclined to engage in behavior that brings them pleasure or the promise of pleasure. Redl and Wineman point out, however, that the effective use of promises and rewards depends on a number of factors: the youngster's ability to relate to the future and delay gratification; the youngster's ability to live up to a contract and "deserve" rewards; the youngster's ability to accept the implications of individual differences (different rewards and different expectations for different children), and so on. All of these abilities are not usually well developed in the aggressive children described by Redl and Wineman.[1]

Punishments and Threats

This technique also relies on the assumption that youngsters will seek both pleasure and the avoidance of pain. From a psychodynamic perspective, punishment is very complex, however, and may raise as many problems as it seems to remediate. For the youngsters with impaired ego functioning whom they served, Redl and Wineman did not view punishment as a viable control technique until later stages of the relationship, if at all.[2]

Threats may be used profitably if expressed in neutral terms as signals of the consequences of behavior ("If you do this, then that will probably happen."). As warnings of punishment about to occur, however, threats are as complex and difficult to implement as the punishments themselves.

The strategies described are meant to handle surface behaviors but they may also be used as part of the effort to "clinically exploit life events." In the next section we see what clinical exploitation of life events means, paying special attention to one particularly useful tool in that domain, the life space interview.

LIFE SPACE INTERVIEWS

The concept of "life space" stems from the work of Kurt Lewin (1951) who noted that behavior (B) was a joint function of personal factors (P) and the perceived environment (E): $B = f(P, E)$. A person's life space then represents the continual interaction between inner and outer forces and equals the individual's psychological world at any given moment.

A life space must be viewed through the eyes of its "owner." The objective realities of the situation are less important than the individual's interpretation or perception of the surrounding environment, because perceptions serve as guides to behavior.

From the psychodynamic view, all behavior is meaningful. The life space interview tries to discover the meaning of specific behaviors by examining the reasoning that led up to them. The assumption here is that if the reasoning process can be understood, then new and more appropriate concluding behaviors can be developed and incorporated into the child's repertoire. The child can learn new ego skills.

Interviewing by appointment, the traditional clinical format, was not viewed by Redl and Wineman as an appropriate tool. Alternatively, life space interviewing is an attempt to help an aggressive youngster focus on feelings and actions and life events as close in time as possible to their actual occurrence. Redl and Wineman have described a number of types of interviews (the "run-in" of outside realities, the "guilt squeeze," the "expressive" interview, etc.) that might be profitably utilized in a life space interview process. Here, we review the two major subdivisions of that process: *emotional first aid* and *clinical exploitation of life events.*

Emotional first aid is the name for the quick action by adults that is necessary to prevent physical and emotional damage to the youngster. It is sometimes necessary to set the stage by using emotional first aid to help the child regain control of his or her impulses before meaningful talk can occur. Specific components might include:

1. *Draining off frustration acidity* by saying something such as, "It's OK to be mad" or "Let's get a drink of water before we talk about it."

2. *Supporting the management of panic, fury, and guilt* by saying, for example, "I can see you feel bad about what happened. Try to calm down and then you can tell me about it."

3. *Maintaining communication,* which includes a variety of efforts to erase blocks to communication. For example this could include setting limits ("You have to stay here with me right now"), changing pace to keep the talk flowing, and reflecting the child's behavior.

4. *Regulating behavioral and social traffic,* which involves helping children remember and follow through on relevant rules and agreements. You might say "Remember we said we'd have to talk about any fights that occurred?"

5. *Umpiring* when it becomes necessary to serve as a judge, issue rulings, and explain the rationale for any conclusions drawn.

Clinical exploitation of life events is simply an elaborate title for the process of extracting every possible therapeutic and educational benefit from a given situation. Contrary to the techniques for the antiseptic manipulation of surface behavior, which sought to stop inappropriate actions in their tracks, the notion of clinical exploitation demands a much deeper effort to turn such behaviors into viable learning situations for the youngster(s) who expressed them. Components include:

1. *Giving a reality rub.* Often, youngsters do not know why they commit aggressive acts nor do they seem to understand the consequences of their behavior. Adults can help youngsters understand their own motivations and contributions to unhappy episodes by "rubbing in" the world's realities ("If you swear at Mrs. K., you're going to be in trouble.").

2. *Removing symptom estrangement.* Feelings and behavior are connected, though the child may not see their relation. Adults must help youngsters understand the meaning of their behavior and the notion that their behavior is purposeful, not random.

3. *Massaging numb value areas.* Sometimes youngsters may demonstrate good values but find inappropriate ways to express them. It is appropriate to say "hello," but hitting people whenever you see them is not.

4. *Selling new tools.* This is an extension of the previous component, massaging numb value areas. Here, the adult's purpose is to help the youngster adopt new and more appropriate methods to express good values or valid feelings. Say, for example, "What's another way you might have said it?" or "It's OK to be angry, but the way you showed your anger made things worse for you. What could you do instead?"

5. *Manipulating the self.* At times, a youngster's aggressive behavior may not have been intended, but was manipulated by the seduction of the group or environment. Here the adult attempts to help youngsters maintain control of their own behavior, even in the face of future temptations.

We can see, then, that life space interviewing deals with both feelings and actions. When well-executed, such an interview can legitimize a troubled youngster's feeling ("You were right to feel angry"), help him or her understand the inappropriateness of the action that followed the feeling ("But it's not OK to try to stab him with your pencil"), and finally, move to the consideration of new behaviors ("What else do you think you could do when you're feeling angry?"). This focus on both feelings and actions should follow real life events as soon as possible so that youngsters can get assistance when they need it most and when it is likely to be most meaningful.

Life space interviewing represents a way in which adults can help youngsters understand the effects of their unconscious thoughts, feelings, and actions on others. It also serves as a model for the application of psychodynamic thinking to the real life situations encountered by educators.

Finally, before ending our discussion of Redl's work with aggressive children and youths, it is important to note two related psychological intervention formats: *milieu therapy* and *psychoeducation*. In both cases, the work of Redl and his colleagues made significant contributions to the creation and development of these two well-known strategies.

MILIEU THERAPY

Redl (1959) defined the "children who hate" in part as the children nobody wanted. They were also the children who seemed most unlikely to profit from the standard clinical treatment at the time: psychotherapy by prearranged appointment. Such children, Redl noted, were far too destructive, had insufficient verbal abilities, and were too here-and-now focused to find much sense in dredging up incidents from the past to be viewed as viable candidates for psychotherapy.

Instead, Redl believed that such youngsters would be much more likely to profit from a total therapeutic environment in which continual efforts were made to maximize each child's psychological growth and development 24 hours a day. Following his work at Pioneer House, which was essentially an experiment in the creation and maintenance of a therapeutic milieu for a particularly difficult population of youngsters, Redl (1959) published some of his own thoughts on the concept of therapeutic environments. In that paper, Redl discussed what he believed to be critical variables in the success of a therapeutic milieu, including social structure, value system, routines and rituals, impact of the group, programmed activities, staff, and others.

According to Newcomer (1980), the life space technique is the critical element of Redl's therapeutic milieu, and it serves to highlight the lessons of the environment:

> Although occasionally the impact of the environment is enough therapy for a given child, more often it takes a trained adult to serve as mediator between the environment and the child. The child's experiences in the therapeutic milieu may go unnoticed if there is not interpretation of those events. Even in an ordinary school environment, an adult's well-thought-out reaction to an event can clarify it for a child and prevent misinterpretation. (p. 326)

PSYCHOEDUCATION

When the principles of a therapeutic milieu are applied to a school setting, the resultant program reflects a psychoeducational model. Here, the educational program derives from the milieu, organized to provide continuous therapeutic benefits to each student. For example, Morse (1974) notes the following important dimensions:

1. Environments must be arranged to reflect the values and attitudes inherent in each child's life space.
2. The teacher is a model for psychosocial identification as well as the more traditional imparter of knowledge.
3. The curriculum is constructed to provide opportunities to incorporate affective learning into the regular school program.
4. The group or peer culture is a focus of educational planning efforts. Helping children learn from their peer groups is of critical importance.
5. The availability of therapeutic resources is arranged and ensured. Adults who work in therapeutic environments (including teachers in the psychoeducational model) need assistance and support from colleagues.

A good example of the development of a psychoeducational program is provided by Fenichel (1966) in his description of the creation of the League School:

> In 1953 the League School started a new kind of treatment facility—one that attempted to keep severely disturbed children within the community by substituting the day treatment school and the home for the mental hospital.
>
> We began with the hypothesis that behavioral changes could be achieved by the use of special educational techniques in a therapeutic setting without individual psychotherapy. This hypothesis was based on the assumption that a properly planned and highly individualized educational program with interdisciplinary clinical participation could result in social and emotional growth as well as in educational achievements. (p. 6)

Fenichel noted that youngsters in the League School needed individualized learning prescriptions based on comprehensive assessments of learning strengths and weaknesses. The role of staff members was to gather the necessary information and use it to build an appropriate educational program for each youngster. Fenichel also addressed the issue of whether psychoeducational programs were primarily psychological (therapeutic) or educational.

We have found that in working with seriously disturbed children the differentiation often made between education and therapy becomes largely a semantic one. A teacher who fosters self-discipline, emotional growth and more effective functioning is doing something therapeutic. Any educational process that helps correct or reduce a child's distorted perceptions, disturbed behavior and disordered thinking and that results in greater mastery of self and one's surroundings is certainly a therapeutic process. (p. 17)

HUMANISTIC INTERVENTIONS

Contrary to early psychodynamic thinking, which was primarily focused on the importance of negative impulses and drives, humanistic psychology represents a more positive model of dynamic thought. Theorists such as Erik Erikson, Erich Fromm, and Abraham Maslow emphasized positive human motivational impulses and the ability of men and women to control negative impulses and increase their prosocial behavior. Thus, humanistic interventions are focused on the enhancement and facilitation of individual growth, self-awareness, social interaction, love, empathy, and so on.

Maslow's (1968) theory of needs is perhaps most representative of humanistic psychology and we describe it briefly here. According to Maslow, all human behavior is aimed at the fulfillment of certain basic human needs. Further, needs may be viewed along a continuum from basic survival needs (food and shelter) to more social needs (love and acceptance) to the ultimate life goal, self-actualization. As the individual matures, higher-level needs usually take on primary importance. Self-actualization cannot occur if needs from lower levels in the hierarchy are not fulfilled, a condition that can cause despondency and alienation. Interventions based on Maslow's theory, then, must focus on helping people recognize their unsatisfied needs and facilitating their fulfillment. Ultimately, successful interventions should have the effect of moving people closer to the realization of their own potential, nearer to the goal of self-actualization.

More generally, humanistic interventions can be characterized by their emphasis on self-discovery and the enhancement of human potential. The client-centered therapy of Carl Rogers, the gestalt therapy of Fritz Perls, the group-dynamics movement (including the early laboratory or training (T) groups, sensitivity groups, encounter groups, and many others) are all examples of applications of humanistic psychology's ideas. Certain of the humanistic interventions are especially relevant to the problems of aggressive youth. For example, Gold (1978) has argued that alternative educational programs may be a useful way to both reduce and prevent delinquent behavior. Gold subscribes to the theory that delinquent acts represent an ego defense against external threats to self-esteem.

There are two important aspects to the Gold position. First, the threat to self-esteem is not necessarily brought from the outside world into school nor is it based on an internal impulse. Instead, the threat to self may arise directly from the realities of school itself. Indeed, Gold points to "failure in the role of student" as the source of much delinquent behavior in schools today.

Second, because he posits that threats to self-esteem stem from the demands of the role of student, Gold suggests that alternative programs with built-in capacities to increase a youngster's success experiences and provide warm and accepting relationships with adults may be the most viable remedy.

The New Model Me

In the same humanistic, esteem-enhancing spirit, Beatty (1977) has reported success in the use of a program called "the New Model Me" in helping adolescents curb aggressive behavior. This curriculum, which includes a variety of values-clarification exercises, situations for discussion, and lessons on decision making, has purportedly been useful even with students identified as having very serious adjustment problems. Based in part on Maslow's theory of needs described earlier, the New Model Me curriculum has eight major goals:

> The curriculum developers worked out eight goals for New Model Me students: understand the human motivations underlying behavior; realize how resources and physical and social environments influence a person's behavior; study the nature and sources of frustrations and seek constructive methods for resolving them; discern that there are many ways to respond to a given situation; determine how constructive their own behavior is; make decisions based on what effects various courses of action will have on themselves and others; understand that aggressive behavior can be constructive or destructive; and use what has been learned about behavior and problem solving in everyday life. (Beatty, 1977, p. 26)

Rudolf Dreikurs and his colleagues have also developed a humanistic psychodynamic approach to the remediation of children's disturbing behavior. According to Dreikurs, Grunwald, and Pepper (1971), all disturbed behavior is goal directed; they identify four major needs that such behavior may seek to gratify:

The child may try to get attention, to put others in his service, since he believes that otherwise he would be lost and worthless. Or he may attempt to prove his power in the belief that only if he can do what he wants and defy adult pressure can he be somebody. Or he may seek revenge, the only means by which he feels significant is to hurt others as he feels hurt by them. Or he may display actual or imagined deficiencies in order to be left alone: as long as nothing is demanded of him, his deficiency, stupidity or inability may not become obvious; that would mean his utter worthlessness.

Whichever of these four goals he adopts, his behavior is based on the conviction that only in this way can he be significant. His goal may occasionally vary with circumstances; he may act to attract attention at one moment, and assert his power or seek revenge at another. He can also use a great variety of techniques to obtain his goal; and, conversely, the same behavior can serve different purposes. (p. 17)

Dreikurs et al. point out that the teaching of discipline ought to be a continuing process instead of an activity to be engaged in only at times of stress. The goal should be to help children develop self-control, not blind obedience to authority.

In order to concretize their approach, Dreikurs et al. offer a number of do's and don'ts of discipline.

Don't:
1. Become preoccupied with your own authority.
2. Nag and scold children.
3. Ask a child to promise anything.
4. Give rewards for good behavior.
5. Find fault with the child.
6. Use different standards for adults and for children.
7. Use threats or intimidation.
8. Be vindictive.

Do:
1. Try to understand the goals of misbehavior.
2. Give clear directions for action.
3. Be future (not past) oriented.
4. Give misbehaving youngsters a choice between stopping their disturbance or leaving the room.
5. Build on the positive and minimize the negative.
6. Try to establish relationships built on trust and respect.
7. Discuss a child's problems at times when both of you are prepared to do so.
8. Use natural consequences instead of punishment.
9. Be consistent.
10. Be honest.

As Gold (1978) mentioned earlier, Dreikurs et al. also call for teachers to provide more opportunities for success experiences if youngsters' antisocial behavior is to be reduced. The key elements in the Dreikurs et al. (1971) system, however, are *natural* and *logical consequences:*

> *Natural consequences* represent the pressure of reality or the natural flow of events without interference of the teacher or parent. The child who refuses to eat will go hungry. The natural consequence of not eating is hunger. The parent stands aside and does not become involved.
> *Logical consequences* are arranged or applied. If the child spills his milk, he must clean it up. In this situation, the consequence is tied to the act. A power-drunk child will only respond to natural consequences; he will respond to logical consequences with rebellion. (p. 80)

Thus, Dreikurs and his colleagues suggest that we have the necessary resources to stop antisocial behavior. If we simply let nature take its course (natural consequences) or help it along on occasion (logical consequences), inappropriate behavior will reduce itself as a result of the distasteful reactions it energizes. Dreikurs et al. note the special problems of adolescents and believe that their approach can help effect a truce of sorts between the warring generations. Unfortunately, for our purposes here, no documentation of the use of natural and logical consequences toward the remediation of aggressive and violent behavior is described.

Reality Therapy

William Glasser's (1969) reality therapy (RT) is another alternative approach that is, however, not easily categorized. Even though some view it as behavioral because of its focus on overt behavior, it also bears considerable resemblance to the rational emotive therapy (RET) of Albert Ellis. It is also dynamic in its emphasis on the development of feelings of responsibility for one's actions and commitment to one's reference group as the goals of intervention. It is humanistic by virtue of its assumption that the failure to gratify the need for love and self-esteem may be the cause of inappropriate behavior.

In order to function effectively in the world, according to Glasser, youngsters need to learn to behave in a realistic, responsible, and morally correct manner. Failure to act in accordance with these principles, he asserts, makes it impossible to satisfy even basic human needs and causes people to feel frustrated and distressed.

Again, like Gold and Dreikurs, Glasser advocates the provision of more success experiences as the way to modify students' antisocial behaviors in school. Reality therapy and the classroom-meeting techniques are strategies to be used for helping students avoid failure (see *Schools Without Failure*, Glasser, 1969), learn responsible behavior, and develop "stakes" in their situations.

Glasser sees schools' adoption of a curriculum that deemphasizes problem solving and thinking as part of the cause of emotional disturbance. He believes that group meetings with their focus on cooperative decision making and social responsibility would make failure less likely and antisocial behavior less frequent in the schools.

Though he has done considerable work with adolescents and has provided much descriptive and anecdotal documentation of the effectiveness of his approach, little in the way of comprehensive analysis of the impact of Glasser's techniques to the problem of aggression in the schools is currently available. Nevertheless, like the other approaches described in this chapter, there is much to reflect on here as we consider the application of psychodynamic and humanistic perspectives to antisocial school behavior.

SUMMARY AND CONCLUSIONS

Although aspects of psychodynamic theory have clearly provided a basis for the development of the productive techniques and strategies described in this chapter, such a viewpoint has also come in for its share of criticisms. For example, the psychodynamic point of view has been criticized because:

1. It presents an extremely pessimistic view of human beings (Newcomer, 1980).
2. Its description of human behavior is based on hypothetical constructs and operations (Newcomer, 1980). Many practitioners have abandoned this hypothetical system in favor of more observable approaches (Reinert, 1976).
3. It emphasizes the examination of the unconscious as the way to mental health despite the lack of evidence for such a position (Newcomer, 1980).
4. Follow-up studies of children who had received psychodynamic treatment have shown a very low success rate (Juul, 1977).
5. Teachers have at times been encouraged to allow the same freedom in the classroom that was practiced in the youngster's therapeutic hours. Such practices created so much aggression and destructiveness that chaos was the result (Juul, 1977).
6. In therapeutic practice, there was a preoccupation with a child's

pathology and limitations and a lack of appreciation for his or her capabilities and strengths (Juul, 1977).
7. There was a tendency to ignore the powerful impact of the environment on a child's behavior. Thus, not enough efforts were made to elicit the support of the significant people in the child's daily life (Juul, 1977).

Although some of the criticisms detailed here are certainly pointed specifically at the psychodynamic model, others (e.g., preoccupation with deficits and little focus on strengths) may be equally valid when applied to other models. Perhaps the most critical problem with the psychodynamic perspective, however, has already been mentioned: the lack of valid and reliable documentation of its effectiveness.

Despite the lack of appropriate statistical evidence, however, there are indications that psychodynamic interventions can work. Gnagey (1968) provides us with the following criteria for judging the effectiveness of control techniques:

> Does the deviant behavior cease?
> Is contagion of the behavior inhibited?
> Are human relations maintained?
> Does learning become more desirable and efficient? (p. 134)

By these, or any other reasonable standards one might choose, it is clear that at least for individual cases, psychodynamic perspectives have demonstrated some effectiveness. Whether they work because they reduce frustration, or activate children's controls, or help youngsters develop stakes in the settings, or build ego skills, or simply impose external authority is less clear. What is clear is that aggression in the American school is widespread and getting worse. The failure to pursue any line of intervention that shows the promise of some of the psychodynamic and humanistic methods described in this chapter would be unconscionable.

NOTES

1. The behavior modification perspective on the use of rewards is presented on pages 86 to 90.
2. The behavior modification perspective on the use of punishment is presented on pages 90 to 105.

CHAPTER 6

Gang-Oriented
Interventions

Delinquent youth gangs in the United States, as a social (or antisocial) phenomenon, ebb and flow in terms of both their numbers and societal impact. As we enter the 1990s, there seem to be more gangs, more gang youth drug involvement, and greater levels of violence being perpetrated by such youth—on the streets and in schools. The present chapter describes the sources and substance of this phenomenon, both in general and in school settings and, with particular focus on gang violence, examines an array of preventative and rehabilitative interventions that have been employed to reduce delinquency and aggression
  The definition of a gang has varied with time and place, with political and economic conditions, with community tolerance with the level and nature of police and citizen concern, with cultural and subcultural traditions and mores, and with media-generated sensationalism or indifference to law-violating youth groups. The answer to "What is a gang?" has varied chronologically from a play group formed out of unconscious pressures and instinctual need (Puffer, 1912), to an interstitial group derived from conflict with others (Thrasher, 1927/1963), to an aggregation called "a gang" via community and then self-labeling processes (Klein, 1971), to singular definitional emphasis on territoriality and delinquent behavior (Gardner, 1983), and, most recently, to a definitional focus on violence and drug involvement (Spergel, Curry, Ross, & Chance, 1989). Spergel et al. (1989) comment with regard to this definitional progression:

Definitions in the 1950s and 1960s were related to issues of etiology as well as based on liberal, social reform assumptions. Definitions in the 1970s and 1980s are more descriptive, emphasize violent and criminal characteristics, and possibly a more conservative philosophy of social control and deterrence (Klein & Maxson, 1989). The most recent trend may be to view gangs as more pathological than functional and to restrict usage of the term to a narrow set of violent and criminal groups. (p. 13)

The contemporary American juvenile gang may have a structured organization, identifiable leadership, territorial identification, continuous association, specific purpose, and engage in illegal behavior—as largely characterizes many of the gangs in California, Illinois and elsewhere as we enter the 1990s (California Youth Gang Task Force, 1981). Or, less characteristically, they may be loosely organized, of changeable leadership, be criminally and not territorially oriented, associate irregularly, pursue amorphous purposes, and engage in not only illegal, but also legal activities. This is true in New York City (New York State Task Force on Juvenile Gangs, 1990). Nevertheless, these groups are more violent and more involved with drugs, and these two characteristics must also be included in establishing an accurate, contemporary definition of "gang" in America.

How else may the nature of delinquent youth gangs in the United States best be clarified Considering causation, that is, asking why gangs form may answer the question. Early theorizing reflected the heavy reliance on Darwinian thinking and used instinct as the core explanatory construct; thus the assertion that one ought to

> look upon the boy's gang as the result of a group of instincts inherited from a distant past. . . . we must suppose that these gang instincts arose in the first place because they were useful once, and that they have been preserved to the present day because they are, on the whole, useful still. (Puffer, 1912, p. 83)

Thrasher (1927/1963) looked for causation both within the youths themselves and the community of which the youth was a part. The typical gang member, in his view, was "a rather healthy, well-adjusted, red-blooded American boy seeking an outlet for normal adolescent drives for adventure and expression" (Hardman, 1967, p. 7). Yet, the youth's environment was equally important to Thrasher. Inadequacies in family functioning, schools, housing, sanitation, employment, and other community characteristics combined to help motivate youth to turn elsewhere—to the gang—for life satisfactions and rewards. This focus on social causation blossomed fully during the next era of gang research, the 1930s and early 1940s, which Hardman (1967) appropriately labeled "the depression studies." It was an era in which social scientists sought explanation for many of America's ills—including delinquent ganging—in "social causation, social failure, social breakdown" (Hardman, 1967, p. 9).

Landesco (1932) emphasized the effects of conflicting immigrant and American cultures. Shaw and McKay (1942) stressed a combination of slum area deterioration, poverty, family dissolution, and organized crime. Tannenbaum (1939) proposed that the gang forms not because of its attractiveness per se, but because "positive sociocultural forces"—family, school, church—that might train a youth into more socially acceptable behaviors are weak or unavailable. Wattenberg and Balistrieri (1950) similarly stressed socioeconomically substandard neighborhoods and lax parental supervision. In the same explanatory spirit, Bogardus (1943), in one of the first west coast gang studies, emphasized the war and war-like climate in America as underpinning the aggressive gangs forming at that time. Dumpson (1949), more multicausal but still contextual in his causative thinking, identified the war, racism, and diverse political and economic sources. While the social problems of the day have over the decades largely formed the basis for explaining why youths form gangs, Miller (1982) has offered a more fully inclusive perspective, which appears to us to more adequately capture the likely complex determinants of gang formation. He observes:

> Youth gangs persist because they are a product of conditions basic to our social order. Among these are a division of labor between the family and the peer group in the socialization of adolescents, and emphasis on masculinity and collective action in the male subculture; a stress on excitement, congregation, and mating in the adolescent subculture; the importance of toughness and smartness in the subcultures of lower-status populations; and the density conditions and territoriality patterns affecting the subcultures of urban and urbanized locales. (p. 320)

DELINQUENT GANG THEORY

The early periods in the history of social science interest in delinquent gangs were thus largely descriptive. What gangs were and the societal/familial conditions that were their antecedents and concomitants were the focus of concern. Little emerged during this time in the way of formal gang theory, that is, conceptualizations of the structural and dynamic variables underlying gang formation, organization, and especially the delinquent behavior that characterized a substantial amount of gang functioning. This theoretical void was filled, and then some,

beginning the in the 1950s. By far the majority of this theory development effort was sociological in nature. It focused primarily on seeking
to explain the delinquent behavior of individuals and groups of youth,
and included the following:

1. *Strain theory,* which emphasized the discrepancy between economic aspiration and opportunity, as well as such discrepancy-induced
reactions as frustration, deprivation, and discontent. Cohen's (1955)
reactance theory, and Cloward and Ohlin's (1960) differential opportunity theory are both elaborations of strain theory.

2. *Subcultural theory,* or *cultural deviance theory,* which holds that
delinquent behavior grows from conformity to the prevailing social
norms experienced by the youth in his or her particular subcultural
group, norms largely at variance with those held by society at large and
including, according to Cohen (1966), gratuitous hostility, group autonomy, intolerance of restraint, short-run hedonism, the seeking of
recognition via antisocial behavior, little interest in planning for long-
term goals, and related behavioral preferences. Sutherland's (1937;
Sutherland & Cressey, 1974) differential association theory, Miller's
(1958) notion of lower class culture as a "generating milieu" for gang
delinquency, differential identification theory (Glaser, 1956), culture
conflict theory (Shaw & McKay, 1942), illicit means theory (Shaw &
McKay, 1942), and what might be termed structural determinism theory (Clarke, 1977) are the major concretizations of subcultural theory.

3. *Control theory.* While both strain and subcultural theories seek
to explain why some youngsters commit delinquent acts, control theory operationalizes its concern with the etiology of delinquency by posit-
ing reasons why some youngsters do not. Everyone, it is assumed, has
a predisposition to commit delinquent acts, and the theory concerns
itself with how individuals learn not to offend, primarily via a process
of social bonding (Hirschi, 1969).

4. *Labeling theory.* In 1938, Tannenbaum described an escalating
process of stigmatization or labeling which he asserted can occur between the delinquent individual or group and the community of which
it is a part. The process of making the criminal, accordingly, is a sequence of tagging, defining, identifying, segregating, describing, em-
phasizing, making conscious and self-conscious. In labeling theory, a
person becomes the thing he or she is described as being.

5. *Radical theory.* Radical theory is a sociopolitical perspective on
crime and delinquency (Abadinsky, 1979; Meier, 1976). Its focus is on
the political meanings and motivations underlying society's definitions
of crime and its control. In this view, crime is a phenomenon largely
created by those who possess wealth and power in the United States.

U.S. laws, it is held, are the laws of the ruling elite, used to subjugate the poor, minorities and the powerless. Thus, the theory holds the social and economic structure of American society as its target for intervention.

CURRENT GANG DEMOGRAPHICS

Data on the number, nature, structure and functioning of delinquent gangs, especially accurate data, are hard to come by. No national agency in the United States has assumed responsibility for the systematic collection and reporting of information about gangs. Each city or region is free to formulate its own definition of "gang," and decide what data to collect. Police — the major source of gang information in most American cities — public service agencies, schools, mass media representatives, and others regularly exposed to gang youth often exaggerate or minimize gang numbers and illegal behaviors as a function of political, financial, or other public relations needs. Compounding the difficulty in obtaining adequate, accurate, objective, and relevant information are gang youths themselves. They have their own reasons, real and imagined, for exaggerating or diminishing the purported size, activities and/or impact of their gang. Thus, we must be cautious in accepting the available data, and conservative in interpreting them. Given these provisos, what do we know now about the structure and demographics of the contemporary delinquent gang?

In 1974, Miller conducted a major, national survey seeking information about gangs from a spectrum of public and private service agencies, police departments, probation offices, courts, juvenile bureaus and similar sources. Particular attention was paid to the six American cities reporting the highest levels of gang activity. Philadelphia and Los Angeles reported the highest proportion of gang members to their respective male adolescent populations (6 per 100). Gang members in the surveyed cities were predominantly male, from 12 to 21 years old; resided in the poorer, usually central-city areas; and came from families at the lower occupational and educational levels. Gang youths were African American ($\frac{1}{2}$), Latino ($\frac{1}{6}$), Asian ($\frac{1}{10}$), and non-Latino white ($\frac{1}{10}$), and had a strong tendency to form ethnically homogeneous gangs.

Needle and Stapleton (1982) surveyed police departments in 60 American cities of various sizes; delinquent youth gangs were no longer seen as a big-city problem. Though the popular mythology is that most such non-big-city gangs are branches intentionally exported by particular big-city gangs or mega-gangs (especially the Crips and Bloods in

Los Angeles), reality appears a bit more complex. While a modest amount of such "franchising," "branching," or "hiving off" may occur, most mid-size and small-city gangs either originate in such locations or are started by nonresident gang members via kinship, alliance, the expansion of turf boundaries, or the movement of gang members' families into new areas (Moore, Vigil, & Garcia, 1983).

By 1989, according to yet another, and particularly extensive, survey conducted by Spergel, Ross, Curry, and Chance (1989), delinquent gangs were located in almost all fifty states. Thirty-five surveyed cities reported a total of 1,439 gangs. California, Illinois, and Florida have substantial gang concentrations. Spergel et al. (1989) report that three jurisdictions have especially high numbers of youth gangs: Los Angeles County (600), Los Angeles City (280), and Chicago (128). Of the total of 120,636 gang members reported to exist in all the surveyed cities combined, 70,000 were estimated to be in Los Angeles County, including 26,000 in Los Angeles, and 12,000 in Chicago.[1] But it was not only these three jurisdictions expressing concern. Spergel et al. (1989) reported that while 14% of their survey's law enforcement respondents and 8% of other respondents believed that the gang situation in their jurisdictions had improved since 1980, 56% of the police, and 68% of the non-law-enforcement respondents claimed their situation had worsened.

Males continue to outnumber female gang members at a ratio of approximately 20 to 1. Gang size is a function of a number of determinants, including density of the youth population in a given geographical or psychological area (i.e., the pool to draw upon), the nature of the gang's activities, police pressures, season of the year, gang recruitment efforts, relevant agency activity, and additional factors (Spergel, 1965). Only 5% or less of gang crime is committed by females. Females join gangs later than do males, and leave them earlier. The age range of gang membership appears to have expanded—now it's from around 9 to 30—as gang involvement in drug dealing has increased. Younger members are often used as lookouts and runners, with the knowledge that if caught, judges and juvenile law tend to be more lenient when the perpetrator is young. Older members tend to remain in the gang as a result of both the profitability of drug dealing, and the paucity of employment opportunities for disadvantaged populations in the legitimate economy. African Americans, Latinos, Asians, and whites are America's gang members.[2]

Why do they join? Largely to obtain what all adolescents appropriately seek—peer friendship, pride, identity development, self-esteem enhancement, excitement, the acquisition of resources, and in response to family and community tradition, goals which are not often available

through legitimate means in the disorganized and low-income environments from which most gang youths come.

How do they leave? They may marry out, age out, and find employment in the legitimate economy. They may shift to individual or
organized crime. Many go to prison. Some die.

What do gangs do? Mostly they just "hang out," engaging in the
diverse interpersonal behaviors characteristic of almost all adolescents.
They may claim and topographically define their territory, make (sometimes extensive) use of graffiti to define their turf, challenge rivals, or
proclaim their gang; they may incorporate distinctive colors or color
combinations within their dress, tatoo their bodies, and make use of
special hand signs as a means of communicating. Sometimes they commit delinquent acts and engage in various of aggressive behavior. While
the absolute amount of such behavior is small, its effect on the chain
of events beginning with the media response, then the public perception of gang youth behavior, and finally of police and public agency
countermeasures is quite substantial.

GANG VIOLENCE

Through the 1970s and 1980s, the levels and forms of gang violence
in the United States have substantially increased, parallel to the levels
and forms of violence elsewhere on the American scene.[3] Whereas the
Roxbury Project (Miller, 1980), Group Guidance Project (Klein, 1971),
and Ladino Hills Project (Klein, 1971) gang intervention programs of
the 1950s and 1960s collectively revealed almost no homicides and only
modest amounts of other types of gang violence, there were 81 gang-
related homicides in Chicago in 1981, 351 such deaths in Los Angeles
in 1980, and over 1,500 in Los Angeles during the 1985–1989 period
(Gott, 1989). Spergel et al. (1989) report that only about 1% of all the
violent crime committed in Chicago was perpetrated by gang members.
The seriousness of such figures, however, resides not only in their relative increase from past years, but also, and especially, in their nature—
primarily homicide and aggravated assault. Such violent offenses, Spergel et al. (1989) observe, are three times more likely to be committed
by gang members than by nongang delinquents, a finding also reported by Friedman (1975) and Tracy (1979). Why do they fight? The reasons appear to be both diverse and complex, and include the qualities
of the world in which the youth live, qualities of the youths themselves,
and immediate, fuse-lighting provocations.

Environmental Qualities

Drugs

To an increasing degree, gang members fight more over drug selling and economic territory and less about turf ownership and physical territory, though the latter still fuel their share of violent incidents. Competition for drug markets, at least in some regions of the United States, appears in fact to be an especially important source of gangs' aggression. This seems to be more the case in U.S. west coast cities, where gangs may have control of the drug business (Spergel et al., 1989), than in east coast cities, in which the drug trade is more likely to be controlled by organized adult crime, and gang youths are assigned more ancillary roles, such as runner, lookout, and the like (New York State Task Force on Juvenile Gangs, 1990).

Territory

The traditional major source of gang violence—territoriality—continues to be a relevant concern. Though enhanced mobility away from one's turf via the use of automobiles, dispersal of many school-age youths to schools out of their home areas as a result of desegregation efforts, and enhanced focus on economic rather than physical territory, have all taken place, many gangs continue to mark, define, claim, protect and fight over their turf. Vigil (1988) quotes one gang youth who makes this point powerfully:

> The only thing we can do is build our own little nation. We know that we have complete control in our community. Its like we're making our stand. . . . We're all brothers and nobody fucks with us. . . . We take pride in our little nation and if any intruders enter, we get panicked because we feel our community is being threatened. The only way is with violence. (p. 131)

Guns

There are 200 million privately owned guns in the United States (Goldstein, 1983), and it has been estimated that 270,000 of them are carried to school every day ("Caught in the Crossfire," 1990). Since 1900, over 750,000 U.S. civilians have been killed by privately owned guns. Each year, there are 200,000 gun related injuries and approximately 20,000 gun related deaths: 3,000 by accident, 7,000 by homicide, 9,000 by suicide. Guns are involved in two out of every three murders, one-third of all robberies, and one-fifth of all aggravated assaults. Such a remarkable level and use of weaponry has major implications for both the level and lethality of gang violence in the United States. The gang rumbles of decades ago, whatever their group or individual expressions, typically involved the use of fists, sticks, bricks, bats, pipes, knives, and an occasional home-made zip gun. The geometric proliferation of often sophisticated (automatic and semi-automatic) guns, and their ready availability have changed matters considerably (Zimring, 1977). Klein and Maxson (1989) put it well:

> Does the ready access to guns explain much of the increase in violence? The notion here is that more weapons yield more shootings; these, in turn, lead to more "hits"; and these, in turn, lead to more retaliations in a series of reciprocal actions defending honor and territory. . . . The theory is that firearms have been the teeth that transform bark into bite. (p. 219)

Gang Member Qualities

Demographics

There appear to be a number of characteristics of contemporary U.S. gang members which, when combined with the environmental enhancers just described, contribute importantly to the increases in gang violence. Two characteristics are straightforwardly demographic: more gangs and older gang members. Both Klein and Maxson (1989) and Spergel et al. (1989) have speculated that these qualities may themselves help account for the apparently heightened levels of gang violence.

Honor

Honor, and its several related qualities — machismo, self-esteem, status, power, heart, rep — long gang members' characteristics purported to contribute importantly to overt aggression,[4] perhaps does so even more so today. But Miller (1982) wonders if honor has become less of a factor in the etiology of gang member aggression. As such aggression has changed in form and frequency from intergang rumbles defending local turf, to individual or small group acts of mugging, robbery or other "gain" or "control" behaviors, perhaps, he asserts, the protection and enhancement of "rep" becomes less focal. We think the opposite. Gardner (1983) has noted in this context, "With few resources available to poor urban young people, a reputation for being tough and a good fighter is one of the only ways to attain status" (p. 27). It is a sad commentary on America's priorities, but we believe that as such

resources have become even scarcer in the years since Gardner's observation, the potential status-enhancing avenues available to our low
income youth have become even fewer. Therefore, youths must seek
such enhancement by illegal or inappropriate means—including overt
aggression.

Sociopathy

One further characteristic of gang members that may be relevant in
seeking to understand increased levels of contemporary gang violence
is sociopathy.[5] The sociopath has been variously described as an individual who is aggressive, reckless, cruel to others, impulsive, superficial, callous, irresponsible, cunning, and self-assured (Magdid &
McKelvey, 1987); one who fails to learn by experience, is unable to form
meaningful relationships, is chronically antisocial, unresponsive to
punishment, unable to experience guilt, is self-centered, and lacks a
moral sense (Gray & Hutchison, 1964); is unreliable, untruthful, shame-
less, shows poor judgment, is highly egocentric (Cleckly, 1964); is unable to show empathy or genuine concern for others, manipulates others
toward satisfying his own needs, shows a glib sophistication and superficial sincerity (Hare, 1976), is loveless and guiltless (McCord & McCord,
1959); and shows a particular deficiency in perspective taking or taking the role of other persons (Gough, 1948). In 1967, Yablonsky asserted that "The violent gang structure recruits its participants from the
more sociopathic youths living in the disorganized slum community."
(p. 189). Reuterman (1975) has similarly observed that "adolescent residents of slum areas who exhibit these traits tend to constitute the membership of violent gangs" (p. 41).

Immediate Provocations

We have examined both the contextual features (drugs, territory,
weapons) and characteristics (number, age, honor, sociopathy) that collectively may function as distal explanations of heightened gang violence in contemporary America. What of its proximal or immediate
causes? What are the common provocations or triggers that spark the
fuse? The following (a 1960 list from the New York City Youth Board)
appears remarkably current. The reader should note that, like the
contextual/youth causal dichotomy we have employed in this chapter,
the Youth Board separately identified "exterior" and "interior" provocations:

Exterior provocations	Interior provocations
Bad looks	Leader power needs
Rumors	Compensation for inadequate
Territorial boundary disputes	self-esteem
Disputes over girls	Acting out to convince self of
Out of neighborhood parties	potency
Drinking	Acting out to obtain group
Narcotics	affection
Ethnic tensions	Acting out to retaliate against
	fantasized aggression

These are, of course, but a sampling of possible provocations to aggression. Moore (Moore et al., 1978) has demonstrated that gang youths are not infrequently hypervigilant in their attention to possible slights, and Dodge and Murphy (1984) have shown that such attention often leads to misperceptions of hostile intent and related misinterpretations of neutral events. As the New York City Youth Board (1960) observes:

> The possibilities [for provocation] are almost limitless since the act itself in many cases is relatively unimportant, but rather is seen in a total context of the past, the present, and the future. Further, the act is seen in a total context of its stated, implied, and imagined meanings, all of which are subject to distortion by the groups, individuals, and the gangs. (p. 69)

GANGS IN SCHOOLS

Events in America's schools are straightforward reflections of events in the larger society of which the school is a part. Though earlier seen and respected as a turf-neutral, truce-governed venue, in recent years gangs, gang violence, gang drug business, and gang gun use have become firmly and broadly established in the American school (Gaustad, 1990; Putka, 1991; Witkin, 1991; Zinsmeister, 1990). Stephens (1992) suggests that the bases for this shift are the opportunity schools provide for gang membership recruitment, drug sales, extortion, and the establishment of protectable turf. Though many schools and school districts are prone to deny the presence of gangs in their locations (often until a major gang incident precludes further denial), Kodluboy and Evenrud (1993) assert:

1. Do you have graffiti on or near your campus? (5 points)
2. Do you have crossed-out graffiti on or near your campus? (10 points)
3. Do your students wear colors, jewelry, clothing, flash hand signals or display other behavior that may be gang related? (10 points)
4. Are drugs available at or near your school? (5 points)
5. Has a significant increase occurred in the number of physical confrontations/stare-downs within the past 12 months in or near your school? (5 points)
6. Are weapons increasingly present in your community? (10 points)
7. Are beepers, pagers, or cellular phones used by your students? (10 points)
8. Have you had a drive-by shooting at or around your school? (15 points)
9. Have you had a "show-by" display of weapons at or around your school? (10 points)
10. Is your truancy rate increasing? (5 points)
11. Are an increasing number of racial incidents occurring in your community or school? (5 points)
12. Does your community have a history of gangs? (10 points)
13. Is there an increasing presence of "informal social groups" with menacing names? (15 points)

Total score
15 points or less: no significant gang problem
20–40 points: emerging gang problem
45–60 points: gang problem present
65 points or more: acute gang problem

FIGURE 6.1. The Gang Assessment Tool. From Stephens (1992, p. 221). Copyright 1992 the National School Safety Center. Reprinted by permission.

Every large urban school district is currently impacted to some degree by street gang activity. The National Youth Gang Survey discerned that 21 large urban areas have a current gang problem and another 24 have an emerging gang problem.... Gangs are present within the boundaries of virtually every major school district in America. (p. 257)

Are there gangs in your school or school district? Stephens (1992) has provided the Gang Assessment Tool shown in Figure 6.1, an informal screening device for providing school personnel with an approximate means of estimating the presence, absence and likelihood of gang development at their own locations.

INTERVENTION

Detached Workers

Gang intervention programming may be described chronologically as shown in Table 6.1. As can be seen, until around 1950, gangs were not a major American phenomenon, so neither were gang intervention ef-

TABLE 6.1. Gang Intervention Programming

Up to 1950: Minimal, unsystematic

1950–1965: Detached work, youth outreach, street gang work

1965–1980: Social and economic opportunities provision

1980–1990: Gangbusting, suppression, incarceration

1990–present: Comprehensive programming: psychological, vocational, recreational,
        familial, educational, criminal justice

forts. As the postwar gang problem grew in the United States, so too did intervention programming—at that time largely in the form of social work procedures to be used by agency staff members who worked, not in offices, but out where the youths themselves were, on the streets. According to Spergel (1965):

> The practice variously labeled detached work, street club, gang work, area work, extension youth work, corner work, etc., is the systematic effort of an agency worker, through social work or treatment techniques within the neighborhood context, to help a group of young people who are described as delinquent or partially delinquent to achieve a conventional adaptation. (p. 22)

> The assumption of youth agencies was that youth gangs were viable or adaptive and could be re-directed. Counseling and group activities could be useful in persuading youth gang members to give up unlawful behavior. The small gang group or subgroup was to be the center of attention of the street worker. (p. 145)

Detached work programs grew from a historical context reaching back to the mid-19th century, in which, as Brace (1872, cited in Bremmer, 1976) reported, charity and church groups—as well as Boy Scouts, Boys' Clubs, YMCA's and settlement houses—sought to establish relationships with and programs for urban youths in trouble or at risk. Thrasher (1927–1963) spoke of similar efforts in 1927, and the Chicago Area Projects of the 1930s (Kobrin, 1959) provided much of the procedural prototype for the youth outreach, detached work programs that emerged in force in the 1950s and 1960s. In the fertile context of the social action movements of mid-century America, many U.S. cities put such programming in place. Their goals were diverse and ambitious. The New York City Youth Board (1960), one of the major early programs (the Street Club Project) during the period, aspired to provide group work and recreation services to youngsters previously unable to use the traditional, existing facilities; the opportunity to make referrals of gang members for necessary treatment . . . the provision of assistance and guidance in the vocational area; and . . . the education of the community to the fact that . . . members of fighting gangs can be redirected into constructive positive paths. (p. 7)

At a more general level, this and many of the detached work programs that soon followed, also held as their broad goals the reduction of antisocial behavior; friendlier relations with other street gangs, increased participation of a democratic nature within the gang; increased responsibility for self-direction among individual gang members, as well as their improved social and personal adjustment; and better relations with the larger community of which the gang was a part.

Most detached work programs, as the movement evolved, came to the view that their main hope was for values transformation, a rechanneling of the youths' beliefs and attitudes — and consequently, they hoped, his or her behavior — in less antisocial and more prosocial directions.

Four major evaluations of the effectiveness of detached worker, gang intervention programming were conducted during this era. The New York City Youth Board Project (New York City Youth Board, 1960), the Roxbury Project in Boston (Miller, 1974), the Chicago Youth Development Project (Mattick & Caplan, 1962), and the Los Angeles Group Guidance Project (Klein, 1968) were evaluated. Each were found to be ineffective. Yet in each instance, while both implementation plans, and later evaluation procedures seem adequate, such was not the case regarding the manner in which worker activities were actually conducted. If this assertion is correct, program effectiveness remains indeterminate, and conclusions regarding outcome efficacy must be suspended. Why do we take this position? There are five reasons:

1. *Failure of program integrity:* the degree to which the intervention as actually implemented corresponded to or followed the intervention program as planned.
2. *Failure of program intensity:* the intervention's amount, level or dosage.
3. *Absence of delinquency-relevant techniques:* lack of direct connectedness between the intervention's procedures and its hoped-for outcome, delinquency reduction.
4. *Failure of program prescriptiveness:* to match technique, worker, and youth in a propitiously differential, tailored or individualized manner.

5. *Failure of program comprehensiveness:* to match the multisource, multilevel nature of delinquency causation with a similarly mult-pronged intervention.

Given these implementation realities, our view of the efficacy of detached work programming must conclude that its demise was premature, and that the relevant evidence, instead of being interpreted as proof of lack of effectiveness, should more parsimoniously be viewed as indeterminate, generally neither adding to nor detracting from a conclusion of effectiveness or ineffectiveness.

Opportunities Provision

Starting in the mid-1960s and continuing to the late 1970s, gang intervention programming shifted away from primary emphasis on the worker–youth relationship and attempts to alter youth behavior by gang reorientation and values transformation, to a greater concern with *system change,* that is, the enhancement of work, school or family opportunity. This shift in gang programming emphasis occurred in, and as part of, the broader context of increased legislation and funding for social programming of many types in the United States during this period. Often described as the era of opportunities provision, Spergel et al. (1989) describe this intervention strategy as

> a series of large scale social resource infusions and efforts to change in-stitutional structures, including schools, job opportunities, political employment . . . in the solution not only of delinquency, but poverty itself. Youth work strategies were regarded as insufficient. Structural strain, lack of resources, and relative deprivation were the key ideas which explained delinquency, including youth gang behavior. The structures of social and economic means rather than the behavior of gangs and individual youth had to be modified. (p. 147)

The proposed relevance of this strategy to gang youth in particular is captured well by Morales (1981):

> The gang is a symptom of certain noxious conditions found in society. These conditions often include low wages, unemployment, lack of recreational opportunities, inadequate schools, poor health, deteriorated housing and other factors contributing to urban decay and slums. (p. 4)

The need for provision of utilitarian and esteem-enhancing opportunity, of course, was apparent as far back as Thrasher's (1927/1963) work and earlier. What was different in the late 1960s and 1970s was America's willingness to respond to such beliefs with a broad program-matic effort. And indeed, many dozens of varied programs followed (see Goldstein, 1991, for a comprehensive summary).

With very few exceptions (e.g., Klein, 1968; Thompson & Jason, 1988) opportunities provision gang programming has not been syste-matically evaluated. We simply do not know whether, or the degree to which, gang youth in general or particular subgroups thereof accept or seek the diverse opportunities provided, nor whether they benefit from them in either proximal, opportunity-specific ways, or more dis-tally in terms of termination of gang membership, committing fewer delinquent acts, and so on. There is no shortage of affirming impres-sionistic and anecdotal support—including a major and highly sugges-tive 45-city survey of both law enforcement and nonlaw enforcement agency views on the effectiveness of opportunity provision and other gang intervention approaches (Spergel et al., 1989). The value of such survey results notwithstanding, the general absence of the rigorous evaluation of opportunities provision gang programming must be em-phasized. Klein's (1968) Ladino Hills Project is an important exception; its careful evaluation sets a standard for future evaluations.

Opportunity Withdrawal and
the Rise of Deterrence/Incarceration

As the 1970s drew to a close, America got tough. A combination of the heavy influx of drugs, growing levels of violence, purported failure of rehabilitative programming, and the rise of political and judicial con-servatism, all combined to usher in the era of deterrence/incarceration, and begin ushering out the provision of social, economic, and educa-tional opportunity. Opportunity provision is not gone, but it is much less frequently the centerpiece of gang intervention programming. So-cial control—surveillance, deterrence, arrest, prosecution, incarceration—has largely replaced social improvement as America's preeminent approach to gang youth.

> A philosophy of increased social opportunity was replaced by growing conservatism. The gang was viewed as evil, a collecting place for sociopaths who were beyond the capacity of most social institutions to redirect or rehabilitate them. Protection of the community became the key goal. (Sper-gel et al., 1989, p. 148)

The deterrence/incarceration strategy came to guide the gang-relevant behavior not only of law enforcement personnel but others' also. In Philadelphia's Crisis Intervention Network program, in Los Angeles' Community Youth Gang Services, and in the other similar gang crisis intervention programs that sprang up across America, the resource worker, who had replaced the detached worker, was in turn replaced by the surveillance/deterrence worker. Working out of radio-dispatched automobiles, and assigned to geographical areas rather than to specific gangs, surveillance/deterrence workers responded to crises, their focus on rumor control, dispute resolution and, most centrally, violence reduction. Maxson and Klein (1983) capture well the essence of this strategy, as they contrast it with the earlier, values transformation approach:

> The transformation model fostered social group work in the streets with empathic and sympathetic orientations toward gang members as well as acceptance of gang misbehavior as far less of a problem than the alienating response of community residents and officials. By contrast, the deterrence model eschews an interest in minor gang predations and concentrates on the major ones, especially homicide. The worker is, in essence, part of a dramatically energized community control mechanism, a "firefighter" with a more balanced eye on the consequences as well as the cause of gang violence. Success is measured first in violence reduction, not in group or individual change. (p. 151)

Comprehensive Programming

Indeed, it is a primary responsibility of society's officialdom to protect its citizens; gang violence in its diverse and often intense forms must be controlled. But much more must be done. Gang youths are *our* youths. They are among us now and, even if periodically incarcerated, most will be among us in the future. We deserve protection from their predations, but they deserve the opportunity to lead satisfying and contributory lives without resorting to individual or group violence. Punishment may be needed, but punishment fails to teach new, alternative ways to reach desired goals. In essence, the implementations of the deterrence/incarceration model may indeed be necessary in today's violence prone America, but they are far from sufficient.

A less unidimensional and more integrative gang intervention model is emerging, one with the potential to replace the deterrence/incarceration model. We term it "the Comprehensive Model,"[6] one which incorporates and seeks to prescriptively apply major features of detached worker, opportunities provision, and social control programming. It is a multimodal, multilevel strategy requiring substantial resources of diverse types, and it must be employed in a coordinated manner for its success to be realized.

We have documented elsewhere the manner in which aggressive and antisocial behavior derives from complex causality and, hence, will yield most readily when approached with interventions of parallel complexity and targeting (Goldstein, 1983). So, too, for gang aggression and antisocial behavior. Both the recent California and the New York State Gang Task Force reports give full philosophical and concrete expression to this comprehensive gang intervention strategy.

The California Report (1981) urges adoption and implementation of a broad array of law enforcement, prosecutorial, correctional, probation/parole, judicial, executive department, legislative, federal agency, local government, school programming, community-based, business and industrial, and media recommendations. The New York Report concurs with this multichannel strategy, and urges further that, whatever the mode, interventions must be preventive, not just rehabilitative, in thrust; seek not only the reduction of antisocial behavior, but also the enhancement of prosocial alternatives; be both comprehensive in their coverage, and coordinated in their implementation; locate themselves in school and other community settings; concern themselves with family, school, employment and recreational domains; seek and be responsive to gang youth input in their planning and conduct; reflect program integrity, intensity and prescriptiveness; recognize that gangs have potential for, and at times actually have, served in a constructive, socially beneficial manner; and be evaluated rigorously.

The desirability of enacting a comprehensive gang intervention strategy in school settings has been both recommended and concretized by Stephens (1992), as well as by ourselves (Goldstein, Apter, & Harootunian, 1984). Stephens urges that intervention efforts, be they for purposes of prevention, rehabilitation and/or suppression, incorporate the combined actions of school, home, police, and community resources. Specifically, he recommends programming which includes:

1. *An in-school gang prevention curriculum,* providing youths beginning in the lower-elementary grades with antigang information. Lopez's (see Stephens, 1993) Mission SOAR program in Los Angeles (Set Objectives, Achieve Results) is a good example. Such programming includes problem-solving training, learning gang resistance techniques, enhancing self-esteem, and enhancing awareness of the negative features of gang membership.

2. *A model dress code,* which prohibits students from wearing any gang clothing, jewelry or paraphernalia, or grooming oneself in a manner that signifies gang membership.

3. *Enhanced understanding of graffiti,* and enhanced use of such understanding for gang prevention and intervention purposes. To paraphrase Stephens (1992), read it, record it, remove it.

4. *A gang crime reporting hotline,* established and employed in such a manner that students, often the best source of gang-relevant information, will find it easy, practical and safe to use.

5. *Support and protection for victims of gang violence,* including debriefing, counseling, and use of school placement adjustments as safety needs warrant.

6. *In-service training of teachers* and other school personnel regarding the signifiers of gang membership, gang prevention and intervention alternatives, and available safety measures.

7. *A visitor screening policy,* to aid in minimizing the presence of nonstudent gang members on school property. Included here are employing security personnel, having identification requirements, maintening a log book, posting signs in appropriate languages and directing visitors to the school office.

8. *Parent notification,* again in appropriate languages, regarding their child's school activity, including any apparent gang involvement, perhaps combined with training parents in skills useful in diverting their children from gang membership.

9. *Community networking,* which seeks to bring together the combined efforts of parents, law enforcement, students, and school personnel in a shared attempt to minimize and counteract gang inroads at school.

10. *A vibrant extracurricular program* providing attractive, youth-oriented alternative programming can be difficult to create and maintain with only limited funds, but has great potential for providing youth with the very resources they too-often seek to obtain via gang membership—self-esteem, a sense of identity, peer companionship, and excitement.

Though the specifics of effective gang intervention programming can and should differ in response to cultural, geographic and other factors, Stephens' idea that programming should be comprehensive, that is, should involve students, teachers, other school personnel, parents, police, and other community figures is one we recommend highly.

Our concurrence with this comprehensive intervention perspective is in evidence in Table 1.2 (presented in Chapter 1). There we listed 126 school violence interventions which have been, or still are employed in the United States. Noteworthy is its multimodal, multitargeted nature. It includes programs and procedures that are student-oriented, teacher oriented, curriculum oriented, and administrative;

that call for physical alteration of the school; or that focus upon parents, security personnel, the community of which the school is a part or, on state and federal interventions. Stephens' recommendations, and our listing just discussed, are best viewed as an incomplete pool of potentially effective programs, to be considered and selected from or used on a prescriptive basis, when they seem to fit a particular school's climate. As Kodluboy and Evenrud (1993) aptly put it:

> When speaking of school-based interventions for youth gangs, it is imperative that the intervention is neither too much nor too little, neither over-reaction nor under-reaction, and more objective than emotional. The role and nature of gang activity within school districts varies greatly across the nation and from generation to generation, albeit, from year to year. A "one size fits all" approach to school-related gang activity is doomed to failure. Any approach which is disproportionate to the actual, measurable, observable impact of gang activity upon a school or community is likely to be counterproductive and prejudicial. An objective, culturally sensitive and prescriptive, data-based approach to youth gang intervention is what is called for when encountering youth gang activity on campus or in the school community. (p. 282)

Finally, in addition to comprehensiveness and prescriptiveness, we assert that gang intervention of whatever type is likely to fail unless gang members themselves are involved in a major and sustained way. An accurate and heuristic understanding of gang structure, motivation, perception, aspiration, and both routine and dramatic behavior cannot be obtained only from the outside looking in. But input from members is not easily acquired. Hagedorn and Macon (1988) observe in this regard that

> we are in the absurd position of having very few first hand studies of, but numerous theoretical speculations about, juvenile gangs. . . . One reason is that the vast majority of sociologists and researchers are white, and gangs today are overwhelmingly minority. (pp. 26–27)

African American, Latino, Asian, and other minority youths do indeed constitute a large portion of America's contemporary gang membership. They bring to their gang participation diverse and often culture-specific membership motivations, perceptions, behaviors, and beliefs. The meaning of aggression; the perception of gang as family; the gang as a status, honor, or "rep" acquisition arena; the gang's duration, cohesiveness, typical and atypical legal and illegal pursuits; its place in the community; and much more about gangs is substantially shaped by cultural traditions and mores. A rich literature exists describing in depth the cultural patterns and perspectives of America's ethnic and racial subgroups—Aftican American (Beverly & Stanback, 1986; Brown, 1978; Glasgow, 1980; Helmreich, 1973; Keiser, 1969; Kochman, 1981; Meltzer, 1980; Silverstein & Krate, 1975; White, 1984), Latino (Horowitz, 1983; Mirande, 1987; Moore, Garcia, Garcia, Cerda, & Valencia, 1978; Quicker, 1983; Ramirez, 1983; Vigil, 1983; Vigil & Long, 1990), Asian (Bloodworth, 1966; Bresler, 1980; Kaplan & Dubro, 1986; Meltzer, 1980; President's Commission on Organized Crime, 1985; Wilson, 1970), and others (Hagedorn & Macon, 1988; Howard & Scott, 1981; Schwartz & Disch, 1970). Especially useful in much of this culture-clarifying literature is the opportunity it collectively provides to view the structure, dynamics, and purposes of delinquent gangs through the cultural lenses of their members, and the support it implies for the necessity of obtaining gang member contributions if programming it to be effective.

SUMMARY

We have described the history of gangs: their demographics, the purposes they serve their members, their activities, and the nature and sources of their frequent aggression in both community and school settings. Intervention efforts have sought values transformation via the widespread use of street gang or detached worker programming, opportunities provision via social infusion programming, and deterrence/incarceration by means of social control, criminal justice procedures. Most promising, in our view, is the period of gang intervention work we may now be entering, that of comprehensive programming.

NOTES

1. This numerical litany of youth participation in gangs should be tempered with the reminder that most youths, even in areas in which gangs are common, do not join gangs. Vigil (1983), for example, estimates that only 4–10% of Chicano youth are affiliated with gangs.

2. Membership strongly tends to continue, and often further solidify, when and if the gang youth is incarcerated (Camp & Camp, 1985; Jacobs, 1974; Lane, 1989). Gott (1989), for example, reports that in 1989 approximately 5,000 of the 9,000 youths incarcerated in California Youth Authority facilities were gang members and that, as others have also observed, gang cohesiveness and activity level appear to be substantially accelerated by and during incarceration.

3. The weight of evidence combines to suggest that delinquent gangs in America are indeed behaving in a more violent manner in recent years (Miller

1990; Short, 1990). Nevertheless, it is important to note that such an apparent increase may derive, at least in part, from artifactual sources. Media interest in youth gangs ebbs and flows, and tends to be accentuated in direct proportion to youth violence levels. The contemporary increase in such behaviors may be partially just such a media interest effect. The likelihood of this possibility is enhanced by a second potential artifact, the relative absence of reliable sources of gang-relevant information. As Klein and Maxson (1989) note: "The 1960s gang programs, which permitted detailed description of gang structure and activity patterns, are now largely absent . . . the current picture is based on evidence that is largely hearsay rather than empirical" (p. 209). Finally, following from the fact that by far the majority of the currently available gang-relevant information comes from police sources, it becomes possible that information regarding increased gang violence is in part also an artifact of more and more intensive, police department gang intelligence unit activity.

    4. Vigil (1988) suggests that fighting with rival gangs is most common among gang members still in their early adolescence, that is, still in their reputation-acquiring stage. Later adolescents, he proposes, are more likely to be initiators of gain-associated criminal activities.

    5. While "sociopathy" is no longer used as an official DSM-III diagnostic category, it remains both a term extant in the criminology literature, and a label communicating trait and behavioral information. Thus, we have elected to employ it here.

    6. It is similar in spirit and, in large measure, its particulars to Spergel et al.'s (1989) model approach.

SYSTEM-ORIENTED
INTERVENTIONS

The Teacher

Given that all the teachers in this study had at least three years of experience and had been recommended as either average or outstanding at dealing with problem students by their principals, the data suggest widespread knowledge and skill deficiencies in these areas. Relatively few teachers had specific knowledge, let alone training, in behavior modification, mental health consultation, or other strategies for dealing with problem students. Many teachers complained of this and stated a desire for such training, but many others stated that their job was to teach and not to act as therapists for students with personality or behavior problems.

— *Brophy and Rohrkemper (1980a, p. 72)*

Schooling can get better only classroom by classroom, teacher by teacher. The teacher's role in the reduction of school violence and aggression is obviously crucial. Just as obviously, the teacher is not the only factor involved—parents, the administration of the school, and the community at large all play a part. But the teacher is often the person at the forefront of any effort to cope successfully with the problem.

Although most disruptive behavior takes place in school corridors, stairwells, and sites outside of the classroom, there are occasions when violence and vandalism occur in the teacher's presence. Often such incidents have been precipitated by verbal insults and threats. While the preceding chapters have described a number of strategies teachers can use to reduce the likelihood of aggression, it is critical that they be aware of the risks involved. When the health and welfare of the teacher and students are at issue, the teacher must seek immediate and additional help.

Teachers themselves have been frequent targets of aggressive acts—51% report having been verbally abused by students; 16% have been threatened with injury, and 7% have been physically attacked (Mansfield, Alexander, & Farris, 1991). It should be no surprise then that when teachers are asked to indicate factors that limit or interfere with their ability to teach, 34% list student disruptive behavior as a major item (Mansfield et al., 1991). This holds for elementary or secondary teachers, but percentages vary somewhat with the location of the school: rural teachers, 29%; town and urban fringe, 31%; city, 43%.

Forty-eight percent of these teachers say the problem of teaching disruptive students is the lack of adequate alternative placements or programs (Mansfield et al., 1991). This response may be interpreted as the inability to remove the "troublemaker" from the teacher's class and/or responsibility, but in the past such placements have not necessarily had positive results. Duke and Meckel (1979) have presented evidence that when the classroom teacher shares or gives up responsibility for discipline to other school personnel, problem behavior increase.

Teaching involves a series of decisions, not all of which are made consciously, but which must be understood if the complexities surrounding the disruptive student in the classroom are to be unraveled. If teachers choose to define teaching so as to exclude dealing with disruptions and violence in the classroom or school, this would result (1) in a severely circumscribed and limited role for teachers, a role which in most modern postindustrial societies has been expanding rather than contracting; and (2) in such a choice becoming, in effect, a forfeit of a decision, because sooner or later every teacher will be involved with some aspect of disruptive aggression in school settings.

Some teachers may regard dealing with violence as the province of police or as the lowering of their status with students (Edgerton, 1977; Foster, 1974). The work of Brophy and Rohrkemper (1980a, 1980b) indicates widespread teacher unpreparedness for dealing effectively with aggression. Their findings are even more striking when one realizes that the teachers they studied were nominated by their principals as outstanding or average in dealing with problem students.

A number of factors are likely to increase a classroom teacher's involvement with aggression. The student population in the United States is projected to become more diverse and, thus, more challenging. Grant and Secada (1990) report the following data regarding students in public schools:

- By the year 2000, 30% to 40% of total school enrollment will be children of color.
- 25% of students are currently poor.

- 20% now come from a single-parent family.
- One in seven students is currently at risk of dropping out of school.

These and other demographic characteristics are even more severe when urban children are analyzed separately. For example, in the largest school districts, currently 70% of the students are of color. This statistic should not be interpreted to mean that children of color will be more violent in school. A complex of characteristics have been found to be correlated with disruptive behavior in school, the worst conditions of which are more likely to be found in U.S. cities. These characteristics include housing quality, family structure, race, population density, and community crime rate (Hellman & Beaton, 1986). All of this suggests that school violence has a complex ecology that should be acknowledged.

While the student population in public schools is becoming increasingly more diverse, the teaching force is projected to become more homogeneous—more white and with a greater proportion of females (Grant & Secada, 1990). This discontinuity between students and teachers has important implications for understanding the social and cultural interactions that come into play in the classroom, particularly as they influence the tangle of processes involving aggression. But there are a number of other aspects of classroom ecology that complicate teaching. According to Doyle (1986) the following are the most relevant:

1. *Multidimensionality.* Every classroom has a large number of events, tasks, performances, abilities, and so forth, which result in choices that are complex.
2. *Simultaneity.* Many things happen at the same time in classrooms. The teacher must attend and respond to different activities occurring simultaneously.
3. *Immediacy.* Events occur in the classroom at a rapid place. Hundreds of exchanges take place between a teacher and students during any given day with little time to deliberate before acting.
4. *Unpredictability.* Classroom events frequently take unexpected turns. Disruptions and distractions are common.
5. *Publicness.* Teachers' acts in the classroom are observed by a large portion of students. Disruptive behavior becomes magnified in such a setting.
6. *History.* A class over a period of time develops a common set of experiences, routines, and norms.

According to Doyle, while their intensity may vary, these features oc-cur in all classrooms and influence the teacher's decision making.

In earlier chapters, we offered a beginning set of strategies to coun-ter the problems of school violence by providing the teacher with use-ful means for its prevention, reduction and replacement. Here we consider teaching from a decision-making perspective, and then exa-mine this perspective as it bears upon the needs of the teacher con-fronted with disruptive behavior in the classroom.

TEACHING AS DECISION MAKING

How do teachers plan, implement, and evaluate the activities that con-stitute instruction in their classrooms, particularly those aimed at minimizing disruptive behavior by their pupils? Teachers may be con-fronted with hundreds, if not thousands, of instructional decisions. (Hunt, 1976; Jackson, 1968). According to Clark and Peterson (1986) several studies show that teachers make one decision every two minutes.

The planning, or preactive, phase of teaching has been given con-siderable attention in teacher-preparation programs for some time, as has the evaluative phase. Preactive decisions revolve around the teacher's planning efforts, and research shows that teacher planning is usually carried out in nonlinear ways (Clark & Peterson, 1986). Teachers may plan in terms of content, activities, student needs, and so on. Evidence has not showed what has been called the rational (linear) model to be the way of experienced teachers. The rational model re-quires the following sequence: (1) specification of objectives, (2) selec-tion of learning activities, (3) organization of learning activities, and (4) specification of evaluation procedures. Whether any other model is better than the rational one has not yet been determined.

More recently, attention has focused on the implementation or in-teractive phase of teaching and the moment-to-moment decisions re-quired of teachers. In Hunt's (1976) words:

> Teachers' adaptation to students is the heart of the teaching learning process, yet it remains poorly understood. It refers to the moment-to-moment shifts in teacher behavior in response to an individual student, a group of students, or an entire class, as well as shifts over a longer per-iod of time. Such adaptation has been called spontaneous, intuitive, im-plicit or interactive. (p. 268)

Calderhead (1984) differentiates teacher decisions as reflective, immedi-ate, and routine. Reflective decisions are for the most part preactive (or even postactive) while immediate and routine decisions are interactive, since they occur face-to-face between the teacher and students. Support for viewing interactive teaching from an information processing perspective comes from Corno (1981). She agrees with Clark and Peterson (1986) that what separates effective teachers from ineffective ones is their ability to simplify information by separating the important from the trivial and by transforming or reconfiguring the information into something meaningful.

Shavelson and Stern (1981) have presented a model of teacher interactive decision making which is described in Figure 7.1. This model conceptualizes interactive teaching as essentially the carrying out of routines. The model in Figure 7.1 assumes that teachers do not consider a large number of alternative routines during their interactive teaching. When students' behaviors fall beyond allowable limits, the model provides for several decisions by the teacher: immediately act, delay action, continue the routine, change teaching routine, and so forth.

Doyle (1979) would encourage teachers early in the school year to establish "automatized" routines in a number of activities. Students can learn these familiar routines and know what to expect. The teacher, in turn, can monitor misbehavior more readily. In his words:

> In view of the frequency and the cost—in terms of reaction time and consequences—of unexpected events, it would seem adaptive and efficient for a teacher to direct conscious processing primarily in discrepancies or anomalies. By specializing in discrepancies, a teacher can anticipate disruptions and reduce the effects of immediacy and unpredictability on task accomplishment. (pp. 62–63)

According to Clark and Dunn (1991), such early routines are thought to persist, setting patterns, limits, expectations and boundaries for teaching and learning for the remainder of the school year.

In a similar vein, some previous studies have suggested that teachers construct mental scripts or images for interactive teaching. These mental pictures of the class describe routines which the teacher monitors automatically by looking for cues that confirm the established procedure. When these cues fall outside the limits of tolerance, the teacher must decide what course of action to take (Joyce, 1978–1979; Morine-Dershimer, 1978–1979). Clark and Peterson (1986) suggest that ineffective teachers process too much information and are unable to simplify this information overload into useful practical decisions. Further evidence indicates that teachers resist changing or interrupting the flow of activity during a lesson. To do so "drastically increases the

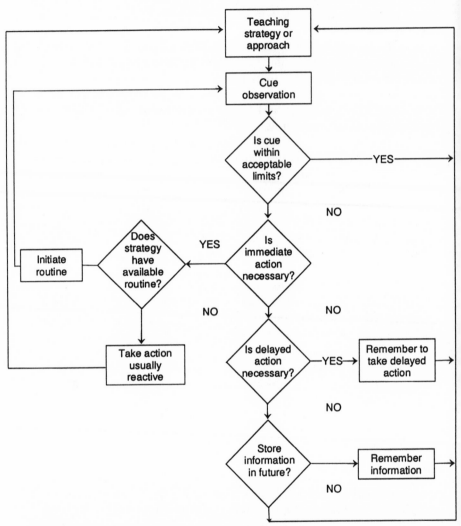

FIGURE 7.1. Model of teachers' decision making during teaching. From Shavelson and Stern (1981, p. 483). Copyright 1981 the American Educational Research Association. Reprinted by permission.

information processing demands on the teacher and increases the probability of classroom management problems" (Shavelson & Stern, 1981, p. 484). Student aggressive behavior constitutes one of the most serious disruptions of the interactive teaching routine and confronts the teacher with the necessity of making a decision. In other words, the evidence suggests that once teachers plan a routine or course of action, they often guard against anything that involves drastically changing it, because such change complicates the classroom routine and makes a successful lesson problematic. If this view of interactive teaching is accurate, the response to student violence in all likelihood frequently involves all of the critical decision-making skills a teacher possesses. The rest of this chapter focuses on identifying those factors which may affect the teacher's planning, interactive, and evaluative decisions about classroom aggression.

PROCESSES IN TEACHER DECISIONS

A number of individuals over the years have presented various views of teachers as decision makers or problem solvers (Bishop & Whitfield, 1972; Clark & Yinger, 1977; Joyce & Harootunian, 1967; Peterson & Clark, 1978; Shavelson, 1973, 1976; Shavelson & Stern, 1981; Shulman & Elstein, 1975). Shavelson has probably developed the most extensive perspective.

Since its original presentation, the model has been enhanced by the specification of a number of factors that contribute to or influence teachers' pedagogical decisions and judgments. These factors are depicted in Figure 7.2. In this figure, Shavelson and Stern (1981) have identified a number of factors involved in teachers' decisions. These factors constitute much of the information the teacher processes. The many arrows in Figure 7.2 between the various factors is an indication that they interact with one another in a number of ways. For example, a teacher's beliefs may influence his or her attributions of student behavior which, in turn, affects how a teacher judges a student and reaches a decision about that student. Taken together, the information in Figures 7.1 and 7.2 present a view of teachers as follows:

> Teachers are seen as active agents with many instructional techniques at their disposal to help students reach some goal. In order to choose from this repertoire, they must integrate a large amount of information about students from a variety of sources. And this information must somehow be combined with their own beliefs and goals, the nature of the instructional task, the constraints of the situation, and so on. (Shavelson & Stern, 1981, p. 472)

What may not be immediately apparent from the figures, or from our comments, is that several alternative decisions are feasible. There is not necessarily one correct decision sequence. Consequently, various teachers who might teach quite differently, but who are equal in

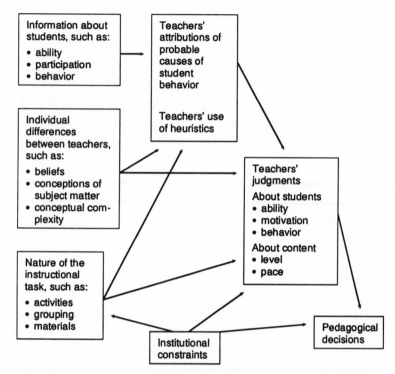

FIGURE 7.2. Some factors in teachers' pedagogical decisions and judgments. From Shavelson and Stern (1981, p. 472). Copyright 1981 the American Educational Research Association. Reprinted by permission.

decision-making skill, might achieve the same goals. The findings of Heil (1960) for example are relevant here. Heil found that different teaching styles yielded very different results with different pupils.

Hunt's (1976) work is in the same spirit as Shavelson's, but has more direct classroom applicability. Hunt's thinking, though not cast in formal decision making terms, has developed out of an information-processing perspective. Let us examine Hunt's approach and see how it can be applied by teachers involved with disruptive students.

Hunt points out that the three salient features of the educational experience are: (1) a student, (2) experiencing an educational approach, with (3) some kind of consequence. Hunt casts these three features into Kurt Lewin's formulation that behavior (educational outcome or consequence) results from the interaction of the person (student) and environment (educational approach). For the teacher, particularly the teacher of disruptive students, the question becomes, what teaching approach with these students will likely bring about the desired outcomes? (Hunt, 1976, 1977).

Hunt (1975) has proposed that at least four features characterize his approach:

(1) it should be *interactive* not only in coordinating person–environment interaction, but in accommodating differential behavioral effects; (2) it should view the person in *developmental* perspective so that differential effects of environmental influence may be seen developmentally as well as contemporaneously; (3) it should consider person-environment interaction in *reciprocal* terms that view the effect of the person on the environment as well as the effect of the environment on the person; and (4) it should consider the *practical* implications of such interactions so that conceptions can be enriched by application. (p. 218)

An interactive approach means that any decision involving alternative courses of action needs to be made in conjunction with consideration of the characteristics of the students involved. The teaching acts or methods must be congruent with the nature of the learners. Interactive in this sense refers not only to the face-to-face instruction between teachers and students, but also to the necessity for responding differently to different student characteristics.

Hunt (1976) has transformed his approach to reflect the teacher's perspective on the process of decision making. Thus, in communicating with a student, the teacher usually (1) begins with an intention, (2) perceives the student, (3) communicates or acts, and (4) checks on the effects. The sequence in teaching may be described as intention–perception–action–evaluation and with the addition of one more step—the teacher's implicit theory about the teaching–learning process—the Hunt model is complete.

The whole process is depicted in Figure 7.3. Hunt's original presentation of the teacher's implicit theory appeared as a step between perception and action (Hunt, 1976, p. 274). We believe the model in Figure 7.3 is a truer representation of what happens in teaching, because all of the processes in teachers' decisions reflect how they view teaching and learning.

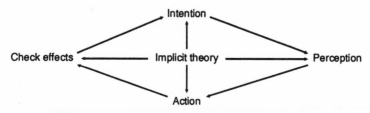

FIGURE 7.3. Teaching sequence for teaching model.

Teachers' intentions, perceptions, actions, and evaluations are influenced by, and in turn influence, their respective implicit theories, which in effect, act as filters through which all other processes are implemented. Although the arrows in this model might suggest a linear sequence, a more dynamic process is likely occurring. Perhaps there should be another set of arrows pointing in the opposite direction to indicate that what is depicted in Figure 7.3 is not static. Let us describe the processes depicted as they apply to the aggressive youngster.

THE TEACHER'S IMPLICIT THEORY

Teachers' personal perspectives of their work have been the source of considerable discussion. More than three decades ago, Travers (1962) concluded that "teachers do not change their ways of behaving simply by being told that learning would proceed with greater efficiency if they behaved differently" (p. 557). More recently Fenstermacher (1979) has presented what he called an "intentionalist" critique of research on teaching. According to this view, "because the beliefs of teachers are not taken into account, any attempt at converting the results of research to rules for effective teaching is essentially 'miseducative' " (p. 20). Harre and Secord (1972) have developed an argument which parallels Fenstermacher's. They believe that "the things that people say about themselves and other people should be taken as seriously as reports of data relevant to phenomena that really exist and which are relevant to the explanation of behavior" (p. 117).

Jackson (1968) has criticized the view of the teacher as a rational decision maker as essentially unrealistic. For Jackson, teaching is an opportunistic process in which the teacher is ultimately concerned about the pupils' learning, but primarily the teacher's attention is on the activities that achieve and maintain student involvement. According to Jackson (1968), teachers focus on the "stylistic qualities of their performance as much as on whether specific goals and objectives are accomplished" (p. 192). Doyle (1979) presented a similar argument and maintains that the teacher's decision priorities revolve around gaining and maintaining cooperation in classroom activities. Doyle has developed a model of teacher decision making based on this perspective. Its importance to the discussion at hand can be seen from the following quotation:

> The analysis of information processing in response to the demands of the classroom underscores the pervasive role of classroom knowledge in teachers' decision making. Understanding the situationally defined task

of teaching and the character of the environment in which that task is accomplished enables a teacher to select activities, interpret events, anticipate consequences, and monitor a system with maximum efficiency. . . . *The present framework, which defines the content of the implicit theories of teachers in terms of cooperation, would seem to offer an appropriate beginning for the study of classroom knowledge.* (pp. 70–71; italics added)

Thus, in Doyle's approach to understanding teaching, the central feature revolves around the teacher's implicit theory of teaching. Moreover, in the case of the disruptive student, the teacher's automatic or routine information processing and attending are interfered with, particularly if the disruption is emotion laden (Doyle, 1979). Cone's (1978) findings support Doyle's approach in identifying the implicit theories of the teacher. Cone found that deviant behavior was perceived to be more disruptive in the whole-class grouping rather than in smaller groupings, and teachers were able to provide elaborate and detailed explanations and suggestions about classroom management and cooperation. These results are consistent with those of Harootunian (1980; Harootunian & Yarger, 1981), who reported that teachers define their success in the classroom not in terms of learning but in terms of the involvement of their students. Student aggression or disruptive behavior was a factor in lack of success for these teachers, but the absence of such behaviors did not define success. Thus, student violence plays a very negative role in teachers' self-appraisal and probably is an integral aspect of their implicit theories. As teachers gain in experience, they view success as (1) increased focus on individual students and less on the group as a whole, (2) an increased repertoire of teaching skills, and (3) greater self-confidence, flexibility, and sensitivity (Harootunian & Yarger, 1981). This last set of findings is in agreement with Doyle's (1979) contention that "beginning teachers are, in effect, simultaneously required to construct classroom knowledge *and* respond to tests of their managerial skill. It is likely, therefore, that classroom demands for beginning teachers are especially intense" (p. 65). The common practice in some schools of putting the new teachers in classes with the most disruptive students simply exacerbates the problem.

Brophy and Rohrkemper (1980a, 1980b) believe that the teacher's implicit theories involve attribution patterns which "form important links in the process that teachers use to construct strategies for coping with problem students, especially when initiating or changing strategies" (1980b, p. 76). They found that teachers' attributions about the motivations and other causal factors underlying simulated problem student behavior are related to their expectations about what they can do to resolve the problem. These expectations also influence the goals that teachers set and the strategies they implement in striving to reach those goals. Recall Brophy and Rohrkemper's (1980b) finding that some teachers thought students engaged in violent behavior intentionally and could control such behavior if they wished. Moreover, these teachers had low expectations for being able to promote change in such students and engaged in strategies involving more punishment, lower-level vocabulary and immediate rather than long-term control techniques.

Hunt (1976, 1987) believes that one of the reasons for inconsistent findings in the study of teacher awareness and its influence on teacher behavior has been the failure to allow teachers to use their own terms in expressing themselves about the teaching–learning process. According to Hunt (1987), to understand which concepts teachers use to view their students, we need to know the content, structure, and malleability of these concepts. For example, the content for Brophy and Rohrkemper's (1980a) teachers regarding disruptive students was largely in terms of controllability and intentionality. Others (Hofer, 1978; Weiner, 1979) have described the dimensions of teacher constructs in terms of ability and effort. Hunt's (1976, 1980) own research has found that teachers define their teaching most frequently in such categories as the student's ability, sociability, motivation, and self-concept.

MAKING THEORIES EXPLICIT

In the earlier sections of this book, we presented a number of approaches that have been developed to help teachers control, reduce, or replace student disruptive behavior. These approaches are based on *explicit* theories or conceptualizations of learning and behavior. In examining these approaches it is important that readers be aware how they differ or converge with their own perspectives. Hunt (1987) has reflected on his own recognition of this difficulty:

> Working as a practical theorist, I became dissatisfied with the conventional view that if a logical theory were developed and verified through research, then it could be directly applied to classroom practice. The abstract idea that "theory led to practice" is logical enough, but it did not offer a satisfactory account of how we were actually working together.... Although I did not understand it clearly at that time, it seems that when both practitioner and theorist identify their experienced knowledge, a sound practical basis for communicating and working together is formed. (pp. 1–2)

To help teachers make their theories of teaching explicit, Hunt (1976, 1980) has used an adaptation of Kelly's (1955) Role Concept

Repertory (or REP) test. Figure 7.4 presents a miniature version of the steps required in the REP test. What we cannot provide is the follow-up discussion of readers' responses, which readers will have to gain for themselves, preferably with a group of other teachers who have also gone through the steps listed.

Teachers and prospective teachers are frequently surprised by both the similarities and the differences in their responses to carrying out the exercise in Figure 7.4. In group sessions that follow, reasons and

---

You need two sheets of paper, six 3 × 5 cards (or similar-sized paper), and something to write with. Here's what to do:

Step 1. At the top of the first sheet, write "About my teaching," and then imagine you are writing to another teacher, someone with whom you feel comfortable. You want to communicate about your teaching so that this teacher will understand how you teach and what is most important in your teaching. Next, write what came to your mind, stopping after five minutes, frustrating as this may be, and turn over the sheet.

Step 2. Turn the second sheet lengthwise, and label three column headings: "Student characteristics" (P), "Objectives" (B), and "Approaches" (E). On the left far side and below the first heading, write 1-2-3 and below this write 4-5-6.

Step 3. After numbering the cards from 1 to 6, write the name (or initials) of six students, one on each card. Select six students who are fairly representative of all your students.

Step 4. Look at cards 1, 2, and 3. "Which *two* of these three students are most alike in some important way and different from the third?" Circle these two numbers on your recording sheet. Next: "How are these two students alike and different from the third?" Write how they are alike as students in a word or phrase under "Student characteristics" (P). Repeat procedure for 4, 5, and 6.

Step 5. Consider those two students circled in the first triad: "How are these two alike in terms of objectives I would have for them?" Record this in the "Objectives" (B) column, and repeat for second pair of circles students.

Step 6. Consider the first pair again: "How are these two students alike in terms of how I would work with them?" Record this in the "Approaches" (E) column, and repeat for the second pair.

Step 7. Look over the three P-B-E entries for the top row (1-2-3). "How are these three features related to one another, i.e., in what way is P related to B and E?" Record below, and repeat for the second row. This requires some time and thought. When you are finished, keep your exercise sheets handy to compare your responses to those of others.

FIGURE 7.4. Steps in making explicit a teacher's implicit theory of teaching and learning. From Hunt (1980, pp. 287–288). Copyright 1980 the College of Education, Ohio State University. Reprinted by permission.

for different combinations of student types and a host of other issues can be discussed and examined.

Figure 7.4 presents but one way of making explicit the teacher's theory of teaching. There are other exercises that might be useful. For example, teachers might be asked to list various kinds of students (students who are hard to understand, whom they dislike, whom they would like to know better, etc.) and then propose objectives for teaching them. Morine-Dershimer (1978–1979) asks teachers to put the names of all of their students on cards and then to group them in as many or as few groups as desired. After completing the sort, the teacher is asked to describe each group's characteristics and explain the similarities within the group, as well as the differences between groups.

Making explicit the teacher's view of learners is particularly important with disruptive students. What teachers believe about students may determine to a considerable extent how they approach them pedagogically. There is evidence that teachers, when provided with knowledge and skills to deal with classroom disruptions, can reduce aggression in the classroom (Borg & Ascione, 1979, 1982; Moles, 1991; Thomas, Becker, & Armstrong, 1968).

It may help clarify matters to consider an example of classroom reality. To understand the teacher sequence in Table 7.3 as it applies to aggression in the classroom, we present the vignette sketched here:

> The teacher is talking quietly with Mary when Don leaves his seat and goes over to Bob's desk, where he begins shouting at Bob, followed quickly by punching him. Bob is not fighting back as much as he is shielding himself from getting injured. The teacher shouts, "Stop!" The fighting continues. The teacher moves closer to Don, grabs his arms, and then removes him to a desk in the corner of the room away from the rest of the class. Don can watch the activities in the class, but there is no interaction with him by the teacher or by any of the other students during the remainder of the time the class is in session that day.

Intention

The adaptation of a teaching approach to a student engaged in fighting must be viewed in the context of the teacher's goals or intent. The teacher first of all has to be able to discriminate and recognize the behaviors that are congruent with his or her intended outcomes. This means that the teacher's intentions must be clear. But how was the teacher's intent related to the response to Don's fighting? Maybe the teacher wanted to help Don learn self-control, or teach Don socially acceptable ways of expressing disagreement and disapproval; or simply to remove Don from interaction with peers for a period time. These different intentions may require different kinds of decisions. The last instance may simply exemplify one of the cease-and-desist techniques that teachers routinely use with disruptive students. But Don's separation from the rest of the class may reflect a conscious decision by the teacher to use nonexclusion time-out (see Chapter 4) as the first phase in a behavior modification sequence. If the goal is for Don to be able to control his own behavior, the teacher may also choose from among the other behavior modification techniques described in Chapter 4. If the teacher views the problem in terms of Don's learning prosocial expressions of behavior, then the subsequent decisions may involve the modeling and role-playing sequences detailed in Chapter 3.

Teacher's intentions can be categorized along a number of dimensions. We have already noted some of these; for example, immediate versus long-term goals. Another important distinction can be made between the teacher's efforts to *prevent* aggression in contrast with how a teacher *intervenes* or *reacts* when disruptions occur. The work of Kounin (1970) is particularly enlightening in this respect. Kounin found that what made a difference between effective and ineffective classroom managers was *not* their ability to handle disruptions but rather their ability to prevent them from taking place. Teachers who planned activities and established rules for behavior were the ones more likely to prevent disruption. Kounin's findings have since been supported by a number of others who have studied both elementary and secondary classrooms (Anderson, Evertson, & Emmer, 1980; Evertson & Emmer, 1982; Partington & Hinchliffe, 1979).

A parallel consideration has to do with whether the teacher's intention is to remediate or compensate for the student's aggressive behavior. Remediation requires that change take place within the student, while compensatory efforts by the teacher or school might control the aggression but leave the student essentially the same. The intent of psychological skills training (described in Chapter 3) is to provide the student with new skills, and it is an example of remediation. Placing the student in a class with fewer students may reduce or compensate for his or her aggressive behavior, but such a move may leave the student essentially unchanged.

When the teacher's intent is clear to both the teacher and to others, the other steps in the decision-making sequence can more readily follow. Moreover, when intent is explicit it becomes possible to differentiate among various intentions, and to match them with appropriate perceptions and actions. The specification of intentions is a skill that teachers can develop (Hunt, 1970). But specifying and distinguishing intentions is only one step in the sequence, and by itself would be inadequate for coping with student aggression.

Perception

The teacher's perception of the student determines to a considerable extent what course of action the teacher will follow with that student or group of students. There is some evidence, for example, that some teachers believe that students like Don who are disruptive and engage in aggressive behavior can *control* their actions and are willfully misbehaving. As a consequence, these teachers have low expectations for promoting stable and global change with these youngsters and use teaching strategies that may be "characterized by a higher frequency of punishment, restricted language, and minimizing of long-term mental health goals in favor of short-term control or desist attempts" (Brophy & Rohrkemper, 1980a, p. 28).

There is considerable variation among teachers' responses in their sensitivity to cues being signaled by the students. According to Hunt (1976), the teacher's perception or "reading" of the student is the priority skill a teacher must have if what follows is to be successful. In the preceding chapters, we described a number of different approaches a teacher might employ with a student like Don. Regardless of which approach the teacher chooses, a "reading" of the student is a fundamental aspect of all of them. Knowledge of the aggressive student is an essential ingredient of psychodynamic and humanistic approaches. For the teacher using behavior modification methods, the issue of what constitutes positive or negative reinforcement for any given student cannot be made without knowledge of that disruptive student. The simplistic notion that teacher praise and attention function as all-purpose positive reinforcers ignores the fact that for some students, including some violent ones, these teacher behaviors may not only be embarrassing, but threatening (Good & Brophy, 1978).

Earlier we noted that the disruptive youngster can be viewed from a contemporaneous and/or a developmental perspective. Knowledge of the student from both perspectives is important, as is the distinction between the two. Decisions made on the basis of the contemporaneous resolution of the student's aggression address the immediate problem; they frequently involve the cease-and-desist techniques which Brophy and Rohrkemper (1980a) noted. Decisions made from a developmental perspective, however, are future oriented and focus on what we expect of the student in terms of growth or change. Both the contemporaneous and developmental perspectives are important, although the former more readily leads to decisions which can be applied to the pressing concerns of classroom practice.

Developmental information about a student or group of students can put an aggression problem in a context that might provide a different perspective for the teacher. For example, in their 4-year longitudinal study, Jessor and Jessor (1977) found that the adolescent who is likely to be a behavior problem is one who does not place much value on academic achievement, has low expectations of academic or school success, seeks independence, and looks at society and its institutions as in conflict with his or her interests. But Jessor and Jessor (1977) note that the descriptors that characterize problem adolescents are the same ones that characterize most youth during adolescence, and they conclude that the "normal course of developmental change in adolescence is in the direction of greater problem-proneness" (p. 238). Brophy and Evertson (1976) also present a developmental perspective for the teacher to consider. As students progress through school, their personal and social development takes them through various stages from being adult-oriented and compliant to being peer-oriented and more difficult to control. The testing of norms and adult values is normal and does not make an overtly aggressive student and, though most teachers would prefer that these behaviors not occur.

It is problematic whether a teacher who understands student development views disruptive and aggressive behavior differently from one who is naive in this respect. There is evidence to suggest that knowledge per se may be a necessary but insufficient prerequisite to competence in making classroom decisions (Glaser, 1981). The fact is, we do not have enough information on teachers' decision making and can only get at it indirectly. Before considering some of this evidence, two quotations, one by Dewey and one by Maslow, are relevant:

> Of what use, educationally speaking, is it to be able to see the end in the beginning? How does it assist us in dealing with the early stages of growth to be able to anticipate its later phases? To see the outcome is to know in what direction the present experience is moving, provided it moves normally and soundly. The far away point, which is of no significance to us simply as far away, becomes of huge importance the moment we take it as defining a present direction of movement. Taken in this way, it is no remote and distant result to be achieved, but a guiding method in dealing with the present. (Dewey, 1902, pp. 12–13)

> This is a ticklish task, for it implies simultaneously that we know what is best for him (since we do not beckon him on in a direction we choose), and also that only he knows what is best for himself in the long run. This means that we must offer only, and rarely force. We must be quite ready, not only to beckon forward, but to respect retreat to lick wounds, to recover strength, to look over the situation from a safe vantage point, or even to regress to a previous mastery or a "lower" delight, so that courage for growth can be regained. (Maslow, 1968, pp. 54–55)

Let us return to our student Don. We have already mentioned some possible course of immediate action that may be appropriate to match the teacher's contemporaneous view of him, such as use of time-out. But what assumptions can we or the teacher make about his developmental level? For example, can we assume that Don has in his behavior repertoire alternative ways of coping with the problem that led instead to his aggression? Do we know what his value system is and what people in his subculture or reference group consider most important? For example, Foster (1974) makes the point that much of what is perceived by the teacher as threatening and illegitimate violence by lower-class children is often nothing more than the testing of the teacher's ability to control and set limits. Of course, Don's aggression has been directed toward another student and must be stopped, but what strategy or teaching act would be an appropriate follow-up depends to a considerable extent on the teacher's "reading" of Don. Again the first step in making inferences about another person is to get information about them. A teacher's lack of information about development particularly when dealing with an aggressive student, increases the likelihood of failure with that student.

The teacher may well note that there are a great many ways that individual differences among students can be viewed. Which characteristics of the individual are most relevant? One of the reasons that Hunt's approach may be of particular value to the teacher is that he has a strategy for identifying student differences that make a difference. In order for a characteristic to be relevant to the practice of teaching, it should indicate a student's susceptibility to different educational environments or ways of teaching. Hunt (1971) has described these student differences as "accessibility characteristics" to which a teacher can "tune in" by implementing different approaches. In other words, the student characteristics that are important are the ones that not only tell a teacher what to look for but what to do as well. The four accessibility channels that Hunt (1971) has identified as most relevant are the student's (1) cognitive orientation, which is linked to the degree of structure in the environment; (2) motivational orientation, which suggests to the teacher the form of feedback and positive reinforcement that is best for the student; (3) values orientation, which identifies the range or context of the values currently acceptable to the student; and (4) sensory orientation, which refers to the sense modalities available to the student.

In the case of the boy fighting in the vignette, Hunt would say that to describe him as a "hostile underachiever" does not provide the teacher with information about how best to approach him. To characterize Don in terms of his IQ is also not very helpful. Knowing that a violent student or group of students have low IQs does not tell the teacher what to do about the violence. Similarly, the student's ethnicity per se is not an accessibility characteristic because in itself it does not say anything about a student's needs. Ethnicity's relation to the functional characteristics of language comprehension or values priorities might provide accessibility information, however (Foster, 1974). Glaser (1972, 1981) has labeled such relevant characteristics as "the new aptitudes" and has urged their study and identification for payoff in classrooms. In Glaser's (1981) words, "teachers and schools need information on individuals that is oriented toward instructional decision rather than prediction" (p. 924).

If future demographic projections describing teacher and student populations hold true, there is every likelihood that teachers and students will come from ever more divergent backgrounds. Differences in race, class, gender, and ethnicity will not diminish. The teacher's knowledge, familiarity and sensitivity in each of these domains may be critical in preventing conflict. For example, Grant and Secada (1990) cite the contradiction between the research finding that effective teachers are the ones who keep the pace of the lesson moving briskly (Brophy, 1986) and the finding by Grant (1989) that many minority students do not participate in lessons in order to indicate resistance. A teacher who has learned only that a brisk lesson pace is the way to teach may run into serious difficulties with a classroom of minority students if unaware of the Grant finding. He or she may attribute the students' behavior to any number of mistaken sources.

In the final analysis, the teacher must make the decisions regarding an aggressive youngster. We present the following questions, the first five of which were originally raised by Ossorio (1973) and supplemented by Hunt (1977) as a guide for making decisions about the student explicit:

1. Who is the person? (identify)
2. What does the person want? (intention)
3. What does the person know? (knowledge)
4. What does the person know how to do? (competence)
5. What is the person trying to do? (action)
6. How is the person trying to do it? (style)

Answers to these questions will better enable the teacher to "read" the disruptive student and proceed to the next decision, even though all of the questions may not be answerable in the context of a specific teaching decision. The important thing is to realize that "reading" a student, particularly a disruptive one, involves knowing the various dimensions involved, and the relations between these dimensions, that describe a whole person. The way a teacher does this is not through a battery of tests and test profiles, although test scores are part of the information, but by questioning, observing, listening, and oftentimes letting the student tell what the problem is. The task is not an easy one in light of the diversity of students that occurs in most classrooms. It may be made more manageable by applying Hunt's (1977) translation of Kluckhohn and Murray's (1949) observation that every student is:

1. Like *all* other students in some ways.
2. Like *some* other students in some ways.
3. Like *no* other students in some ways.

These three statements enable the teacher to sometimes teach and adapt the teaching to an entire class, sometimes to smaller groups within a class, and sometimes to an individual student. For most teachers, these three levels reflect what they do intuitively; the difference once again has to do with conscious decisions on the part of the teacher, more so when those decisions focus on the aggressive or disruptive student. Adaptation to individual differences becomes feasible once the teacher decides at what level it is going to occur. Even if it takes place only at the second level, such adaptation provides an initial response to *some* of the student's uniqueness. Let us now consider the process by which teachers decide to implement action, a process which may occur simultaneously with the "reading" of the student.

Action

In considering the alternative courses of action the teacher might utilize, we need to differentiate more specifically the various levels at which an action may be planned and implemented. The teacher may engage in (1) a specific teaching act, (2) a sequence of teaching acts, or (3) macroteaching methods. For the behavior problem depicted in the vignette earlier, the specific teaching acts include restraining Don and removing him from the group to a time-out location in the class; the sequence of acts may include ignoring (see Chapter 4), time-out (see Chapter 4), and response cost (see Chapter 4); and the macroteaching methods or strategies might engage him in the series of structured learning activities (outlined in Chapter 3) whose aim is to teach Don and classmates prosocial behaviors which are based on a particular model of teaching and learning.

It is the action within the classroom that most people regard as the essence of teaching. For Gump (1982) the action structure is the heart of the classroom. As classrooms are currently organized, the teacher's task is to manage the group. Aggression, however, is usually manifested by one or two students initially. Thus, while we focus on the individual as the aggressor, the fact that teaching takes place within a group must be kept in mind. The teacher must maintain a balance between strategies for coping successfully with both group and individual outcomes.

Hunt (1976) regards "reading" and "flexing" as the essential actions which constitute teaching. Flexing or responding to students may occur over a brief period and then be repeated with changes required by the information the teacher has "read." These moment-to-moment multiple teaching transactions are microadaptations, whereas the various approaches we have presented are macroadaptations. The important point about the latter is that they serve in one sense as a strategy the teacher may use to derive the microadaptations or decisions. In other words, if a teacher consciously makes a decision to work within the framework of a particular approach, then many moment-to-moment decisions have to be carried out consistently with a specific direction; otherwise the macroteaching method becomes moot. The conscious choice of a macrostrategy also will make the teacher aware of, and perhaps facilitate, the teacher's planning, interactive, and evaluative options about the disruptive student.

What little evidence there is suggests that teachers vary considerably in their ability to implement alternatives. A teacher's plans may considerably affect what options are available: *"In effect the selection of materials and the subsequent activity flow established the 'problem frame'—the boundaries within which decision making will be carried on"* (Joyce, 1978–1979, p. 75; italics in the original).

Wang and Walberg (1991) in their review of over 200 recent studies on teaching effectiveness have identified an "important constellation of variables." Included are the degree of cooperativness, goal-directedness and cohesiveness in classrooms; whether or not a variety of educational approaches and activities is used; whether systematic sequencing of instruction is employed; whether direct as well as cooperative group learning is used, and time on task.

More specifically, effective action by the teacher would appear to require lessons that have been thoughtfully planned, reflect established classroom norms for behavior, and minimize interruptions. The teacher's actions demonstrate awareness of what is going on by closely monitoring activities and dealing with distractions and disruptions before they escalate. Effective action requires the teacher to set an appropriate pace for a lesson and to make smooth transitions from one segment to another.

The actions a teacher will take will depend on what is available from the teacher's repertoire of skills and strategies. For example, a teacher who is experienced and comfortable in using cooperative learning approaches (Johnson & Johnson, 1988) may decide to use this strategy with Don. By placing Don in a cooperative group that includes a peer who is not violent but is like Don in most other respects, the teacher might be able to provide Don with an appropriate model of behavior as well a source of support (Williams, Meyer, & Harootunian, 1992).

The question remains how the teacher might develop expertise in responding rapidly and without much conscious deliberation to the problems of violent and disruptive students. By extrapolating from studies of expertise in other areas (Chase & Simon, 1973; Glaser, 1981; Larkin, McDermott, Simon, & Simon, 1980), we can say that expert teachers need to develop a large repertoire of specific "reading" and "flexing" patterns that can be accessed in their memory and quickly recognized. Expert teachers would organize their knowledge of disruption and violence around the central principles explicated in this book. As Glaser (1981) notes:

> In general, then, the learning and experience of the competent individual results in knowledge and in an organization of that knowledge into a fast-access pattern recognition or encoding system that greatly reduces the mental processing load. Understanding appears to result from these acquired knowledge patterns that enable an individual to form a particular representation of a problem situation. Novices have systematic knowledge structures at a qualitatively different level than do experts, and the relative adequacy of the initial representation of a situation (which is determined by acquired knowledge structures) appears to be an index of developing competence. (p. 932)

Consistent with Glaser's argument, there is evidence to suggest that expertise in teaching follows a similar pattern. Novice teachers, even novices with strong academic backgrounds, "read classrooms" and students more naively than those with more opportunity and experience to develop expertise (Berliner, 1988; Sabers, Cushing, & Berliner, 1991). Berliner (1988) has characterized these differences in teaching expertise by identifying five developmental stages: novice, advanced beginner, competent, proficient, and expert.

We began this chapter with a quotation from Brophy and Rohrkemper (1980a), who found that few of their teachers, irrespective of their experience, were able to deal adequately with aggressive students even though the information about how to help such students is available. Whether possession of that information would result in better teaching performance is not clear, but without such knowledge, teachers' roles in addressing the difficulties with disruptive individuals will most likely continue to be less than competent.

Check Effects

The teacher's adaptation to students is a dynamic process. This simply means that teachers monitor and adapt their activities on a continuing basis. Adaptation cannot be a static, one-shot process that responds to the student inflexibly. The teacher's evaluation of the effects of responses to a disruptive incident is the last phase of one teaching act and the beginning of another. The sequence that ends with the evaluation phase of the decision process may occur in a brief time period or it may take place over a longer interval. Let us look again at the sequence depicted in Figure 7.1. Each of the diamond-shaped items represents a decision requiring evaluative activity by the teacher. The sequence is repeated with the appropriate readjustments imposed by the disparity between intention and evaluation. Going back to Don, our fighting student, whether the time-out strategy is the way to deal with him will depend on his responses to it. If he is unresponsive in terms of controlling his immediate aggression, other steps might be taken. The long-term strategy with respect to Don and others like him will similarly be evaluated in terms of their specific behavioral consequences.

Checking the effects of attempts to ameliorate aggressive behavior necessitates going beyond the usual cognitive outcomes or products utilized by most schools. Current calls for alternative forms of evaluation such as authentic assessment or performance assessment still focus largely on cognitive criteria. The effects of interventions for aggression control, prevention, reduction, and replacement will more likely be concerned with process variables like anger control, acceptable ways of expressing disagreement, dealing with frustration, and so on. Assessing such outcomes is more complex, but teachers (and students) can be very creative in designing ways to determine the effects of their efforts. Authentic assessment portfolios for disruptive students might include baseline data, positive and negative examples of group participation, competitive behavior, cooperative behavior, and the like. Most importantly, such a record will focus on the student's actual performance and goal attainment. The teacher is in the best position to collect various samples of the student's actions over time and over many situations.

TEACHERS AS PEOPLE: PRACTICAL CONSIDERATIONS

In this chapter we have focused on the teacher's decisions about disruptive, violent students as if these decisions take place in a logical sequence. Of course, in the real world of teaching, many of these decisions are made in microseconds, and the sequence often is not precisely as we have depicted it. Until the development of an alternative decision sequence that fits the real world better, however, we think our depiction is helpful to those who would improve in their working with youngsters who manifest overt aggression. We have looked at the tasks and activities of teaching without venturing into the nature of schools or the context of the community in which a school is located, because we address these facets in the chapters which follow. We want to stress now that teachers are persons who represent a good portion of the range of human strengths and foibles. Like everyone else, teachers have needs and concerns, and paramount among them, as consistently revealed by recent Gallup polls, has been the question of discipline. Even though the school may stress that teaching basic skills and subject matter is its primary task, a secondary goal has always been the development of responsible and social behavior. For teachers, these priorities are reversed because teachers know that if hostility and aggression are not ameliorated, the first set of priorities becomes moot.

The teacher is not "Superman" or "Superwoman." There are individuals in the class who need more help than the teacher alone can provide. Various services (e.g., resource teachers, school psychologists, school social workers) are available, and they can provide assistance to the student, the student's family, and the teacher. The problem is that teachers usually wait until youngsters' antisocial behaviors have become well established before responding. Longitudinal studies of disruptive youngsters indicate that teachers' assessments of antisocial behavior can predict these behaviors in children up to 9 years after the original assessment (Feldhusen, Roeser, & Thurston, 1977). Awareness of a problem is only the first step in any problem-solving process, but it is the crucial one.

Dealing with aggression in the classroom is one of the most difficult tasks that confronts a teacher. It requires both strength and sensitivity on the part of the teacher, two qualities which apparently are independent of one another (Hunt, 1971). Strength is determined by how well a teacher can control and regulate disruptive students, whereas sensitivity is reflected in the teacher's perception of the cues signaled by these students. The teacher's acquisition of these characteristics is what this book is all about. Of course, there are other qualities or characteristics that would help, but we must be careful in listing them so that we do not end up with a description of the ideal human being rather than an effective teacher, for whom characteristics like friendliness, emotional maturity, sincerity, and so on are important. The personal qualities that make a teacher a good decision maker would likely involve the ability to (1) remain calm in crisis situations; (2) listen actively and not become defensive or authoritarian; (3) avoid win–lose situations; and (4) "maintain a problem-solving orientation rather than resort to withdrawal, blaming, or hysteria, or other emotional overreactions" (Brophy & Putnam, 1979).

Like most skills, decision-making skills in teaching require practice or experience for improvement. There is a growing body of evidence (Fuller & Bown, 1975; Harootunian & Yarger, 1981; Berliner, 1988) that teachers go through developmental stages with respect to their teaching. The facility with which decisions about violent behavior are made will reflect in part a teacher's particular developmental status. Of course, no two teachers, classrooms, and contexts of violence can ever be precisely the same, but paraphrasing an earlier quotation from Hunt, we point out that every teacher is:

1. Like all other teachers in some decisions.
2. Like some other teachers in some decisions.
3. Like no other teachers in some decisions.

Conscious decision making requires more thoughtful teaching and is hard work. No one claims it will be easy, especially in the face of aggression.

The School

The American school, which just a few decades ago was looked upon as a key to solving many of society's problems, has become one of the problems. The public's perception of school has changed from one that supports the claim that "education prevents delinquency" to the belief that "schools create rather than prevent delinquency and discipline problems" (Duke, 1978a, p. 425).

We think school aggression is attributable in part to an inadequate conceptualization of the problem; furthermore, we think it involves complex and multiple variables and cannot be dealt with meaningfully and effectively without similar complex and multiple interventions. (Harootunian & Apter, 1983; Goldstein, Apter, & Harootunian, 1984; Zwier & Vaughan, 1984; Harootunian, 1986). This perspective of school aggression may be called the ecological, interactionist, or systems approach. Accordingly, aggression will be countered most readily when interventions consider simultaneously the disruptive youngsters, their teachers, the school's administrators, and out-of-school variables such as parents and community.

An approach by Wenk (1975) to the school aggression problem, while multifaceted, would require the complete restructuring of the public school system. He believes that schools as currently structured fail to provide students sufficient opportunity to develop into responsible citizens. To make the schools more responsive to all of their students, Wenk has proposed a continuum of five levels of strategies for school programs as follows:

Primary action: an a priori education and human services model to improve the lives of students.

Primary prevention: a strategy that is aimed at children in need who are not necessarily "delinquency prone." The focus is on providing help to the youngster who requires it and not on delinquency prevention per se.

Prevention: a program that focuses on individual children who are likely to become deviant. These children are "targeted" as delinquency prone.

Treatment or sanctions: a strategy aimed at youngsters manifesting inappropriate or maladaptive behaviors that have become unacceptable and have elicited responses from school or community authorities and in all likelihood will involve the criminal justice system.

Rehabilitation and correction: a strategy addressing delinquents who have returned to the school on probation or parole. (p. 8)

Wenk's approach is important because it provides schools with a comprehensive and integrated set of programs. Unfortunately, it has not been fully implemented, but it does provide schools with a long-range blueprint of what is possible.

Another approach has been developed by Duke (1980) through his Systematic Management Plan for School Discipline. Duke maintains that schools can deal with behavior problems by acknowledging that a school is made up of interdependent units. Schools need to make sure that each of these organizational units is functioning properly and is related to the others. Of particular importance in Duke's model are school rules and sanctions, school records and information processing, conflict resolution methods, trouble-shooting mechanisms, community involvement, environmental design, and staff development. To implement Duke's model, a three-phase process is presented: (1) preliminary assessment, (2) planning and enactment of the plan, and (3) review and revision. The strategy involves much deliberation and participation in order to effect changes that would reduce disruptive behavior.

At a general level, we know how to create positive school experiences for aggressive youngsters, and we have known for quite some time. Translating the generalities into classroom environments and organizational policies is more challenging. Currently there is no shortage of approaches for the control of violence and vandalism. Most of these have worked in some places at various times, but they may be best described as a piecemeal.

Another difficulty is that school aggression is seen too often as someone else's responsibility. Scapegoating and blaming are frequently the consequence of such perceptions among teachers, students, administrators, parents, school boards, and in society at large—all of whom blame each other (McPartland & McDill, 1977). These diverse views are reflected in the scholarly literature on school aggression. Stinchcombe (1964) has attributed disruptive behavior to the elitist character of the school. Others have explained violence and vandalism by their descriptions of schools as promoting competitive individualistic values (Sexton, 1967), "mindlessness" (Silberman, 1970), restrictive of achievement opportunity (Cullen & Tinto, 1975), fostering of "immorality" (West, 1975), bureaucratic (Duke, 1976), and even more severe terms. Probably all of these descriptions are valid in some form, and the contribution of the school itself to violence and vandalism will continue to be a matter of controversy and conjecture.

The school uniquely is the institution where the forces bearing upon the behavior of youth all come together. On entering school, youngsters reflect the influence of their families and the social, psychological, economic, and political environments in which their development has taken place. The school may help the youngsters solve or at least cope with the problems resulting from these environments, or it may even create new ones (Glasser, 1969). The school acting alone probably will have difficulty ameliorating the problem of violence, but the school is the crucial agent. Other agencies and institutions have neither the opportunity nor the focus and concentration of youth that the school has.

THE ROLE OF THE SCHOOL

Does that school provoke or ameliorate aggressive behavior? There is considerable controversy over the answer to this question. Gold (1978) maintains that the school controls "the major social psychological forces that generate delinquency" (p. 290) and consequently is a significant provoker of delinquent behavior. Gold's argument is consistent with the findings of Elliott and Voss (1974), who conducted a longitudinal study of school behavior and its relationship to delinquency and dropout. They claim that "the school is the critical generating milieu for delinquency" (p. 203), because it creates in one setting all of the necessary conditions for aggressive or disruptive behavior. Youngsters do not arrive at school categorized as failures or successes, but the school soon identifies them as such and makes their failure obvious to themselves and others. Delinquent or disruptive behavior in school is a face-saving way of defending themselves from such humiliations.

As a result of their longitudinal research, Polk and Schaeffer (1972) attributed delinquent and violent behavior to the way in which schools operate within their organizational structure. They argue that particularly with respect to students from low-income families, the way most American schools are organized guarantees that some students will fail and that some will be discipline problems. In sum, Polk and Schaeffer believe that a youngster's commitment to violent behavior is largely a consequence of negative school experiences.

The finding (Elliott & Voss, 1974) that dropouts had a higher rate of police contacts while in school than did graduates, but that their police contacts declined to a lower rate than that of graduates after they dropped out of school, is one of the crucial pieces of evidence presented by those who regard the school as a contributor to the violence problem. The research of Frease (1973) and Kelly (1975) on tracking systems used in secondary schools also suggests that organizational structures, such as tracking, used by educational institutions may contribute to the incidence of disruptive and delinquent behavior. Frease (1973) reported that youngsters in low academic tracks become increasingly dissatisfied with, and less committed to, school and develop more associations with peers who are predelinquent or delinquent. Kelly (1975) found that tracking position was the best predictor of delinquent behavior when the effects of such variables as achievement in school, sex, and socioeconomic status were controlled. Simply stated, those who maintain that the school is the main cause of disruptive behavior argue that upon entering school children become labeled as "losers" by teachers, administrators, and other youngsters, and end up fulfilling that expectation.

But others who have examined the problem of school violence believe that the school, though it is an important factor, is not the principal source of disruption and delinquency. McPartland and McDill (1977) concluded that the school, even though it contributes to student aggression, is not the source of the problem. Feldhusen and his colleagues agree with this view (Feldhusen, Aversano, & Thurston, 1976; Feldhusen, Roeser, & Thurston, 1977; Feldhusen, Thurston, & Benning, 1973). They collected and analyzed longitudinal data on more than 1,500 children who could be categorized as exhibiting prosocial or disruptive behavior in grades three, six, or nine. The youngsters were followed for eleven years through extensive testing, parental interviews, and behavioral measures. Feldhusen and his associates found that school-related factors were not as important as family variables in differentiating the prosocial and aggressive children. They also report that variables such as the original teachers' assessments of behavior and IQ can predict delinquency over the long term with considerable accuracy.

Another view of the role of schools comes from the Bayh Subcommittee Report (Bayh, 1977). Gangs use schools as their base of operations and recruiting. Drug sales, extortion, robberies, and meetings all take place within the school, especially in big-city schools. Much of the vandalism and violence by these gangs is not for material gain (McPartland & McDill, 1977) and may reflect the extension of street-corner norms and behavior into the school (Foster, 1974). Neill (1978) believes that gangs are at the root of fear among teachers and students. Gangs may be the most serious problem confronting big-city schools.

The school's role in relation to gangs may be described as providing an accessible target of opportunity—opportunity to carry out all of the gangs' activities with relatively little risk. But this role obviously makes the school a victim rather than a provoker of violence as noted earlier. More importantly, violence and aggression are not the exclusive province of low-income, inner-city, or minority students. As the data in Chapter 1 show, the increase in school-related aggressive behavior has occurred in urban, suburban, and rural schools—schools in which gangs are not always easy to find.

Wenk (1975) provides yet another perspective on the school's contribution to school violence. He attributes the increase in disruptive behavior across all schools as a reflection of the disparity between society's greater complexity and instability and the school's maintenance of programs intended for and geared to a simpler, more predictable world. In sections that follow we consider some of the options posited by Wenk and others to counter school violence. We stress here that no matter how the school's role is viewed with regard to causation, all agree that schools play a central role regarding intervention for violent and disruptive behavior by youth.

PROGRAMS FOR PREVENTION, REDUCTION, AND REMEDIATION

Every school wants to counter violence and vandalism, and there is no lack of suggested ways to do that. In some school districts, there are more programs than schools. Los Angeles in 1977 was reported to have more than 40 programs to combat school aggression (Marvin, McCann, Connolly, Temkin, & Henning, 1977). In Chapter 1 we listed 126 programs designed to prevent or reduce school violence and vandalism in the United States. A few examples of programs available to school personnel are sufficient to illustrate both their number and variety.

Many of the solutions focus on security measures or changes in the physical structure of the school. Rascon (1981) would use security officers to reduce aggressive actions. Harris (1981) suggests that the installation of a computer system to monitor fire, burglary, and vandalism would not only reduce crime, but energy costs as well. Falk and Coletti (1982) report on reduced vandalism by the addition of low-pressure sodium lighting. Smith (1982) presents a number of strategies for stronger school security including restricted access to keys, an after-hours alarm system, and full prosecution of vandals. Lewis (1982) cites silent alarm systems, visits to the school at odd hours by the principal, quick repair of broken equipment, and other suggestions as ways of reducing vandalism. Mancuso (1983) presents a similar list of steps that can be taken by schools.

A number of behavioral approaches have been described and recommended as ways of curbing school-based aggression. DeJames (1981), McCormack (1981), White and Fallis (1981), and Bullock (1983) all describe programs that focus on the use of rewards or such behavior-change strategies as response cost and time-out. Some of these programs are aimed at elementary, as well as the usual secondary school students.

In their survey of such school programs, Marvin and his colleagues (Marvin et al., 1977) found that (1) each of these programs is tailored to the individual needs of the particular school; (2) many different approaches have been attempted; (3) many of these programs seem to reduce violence and disruption in the schools; and (4) one of the major factors in the successful reduction of school violence appears to be close cooperation among school personnel, outside community agencies, parents, students, and the community at large. This last finding is essentially the approach advocated in this volume.

A factor not identified by Marvin et al. (1977), and one that might be a crucial antecedent to any successful program to counter school violence, may be the explicit admission that violent behavior is a problem in the school. In other words, schools that initiate a specific program to reduce disruptive and aggressive behavior by taking this step have acknowledged and defined a problem that needs attention. It may well be that the reason most programs designed to reduce school violence are reported as successes is less a matter of what they do than a result of the fact that they do something.

Duke's (1978b) survey of 100 randomly selected high schools in New York and 100 in California adds support to this thesis. In both states, urban and non urban high school administrators identified their three most severe discipline problems as skipping class, truancy, and lateness to class. Duke presents some data that teachers, on the other hand, identify classroom disruption, fighting, and disrespect for teacher authority as the most pressing problem. Interestingly administrators ranked fighting, disruption, drug use, and profanity among the least important discipline problems in school. Duke speculates that students would rate theft and fighting as their most serious problems and notes the following:

> If my speculations concerning teacher and student perceptions of the most pressing discipline problems are accurate, it becomes somewhat more understandable why a "crisis" in school discipline seems to exist. *Each of the three major role groups involved in high schools is concerned primarily about a different set of discipline problems.* Self-interest dictates priorities. (Duke, 1978b, p. 326; italics in the original)

Thus, the perception of the problem of school violence may not necessarily be shared by its various constituencies. Resolving the differences and clearly defining the problem may be the first, and most important, step in reducing school disruptions. In this concept, the principal's influence on the behavior and attitudes of staff are well documented (Rutherford, 1985; Sweeney, 1982). A principal who wants to facilitate positive efforts for all children may have a very hard time doing so, but a principal who doesn't care, or is hostile, will undoubtedly fail. The adults in schools must focus on their interrelationships. They must cooperate, coordinate, give and receive feedback, change some of their own time-honored behaviors, and generally be willing to change first—not wait for children to change. Some stumbling blocks are gossip, negativism, and reliance on only child-focused strategies. Principals are in a position of power to promote cooperation among teachers instead of competition, and to give feedback that builds teacher skills and increase their confidence in dealing with difficult problems.

In sum, how something becomes part of a school's way of doing things is largely a reflection of its principal. There is much evidence both in the United States and Great Britain that supports the position that what a principal or head of a school does affects the social–psychological climate in that school. The climate, in turn, influences not only the academic accomplishments of the students but the incidence of delinquent behavior as well (Rutter, Maughan, Mortimore, & Ouston, 1979; Wynne, 1980). To put is simply, for the fortunate school the problems of violence and vandalism are often on their way to being solved by the appointment of the right person as principal.

The examples in this section are adequate to underscore the point that most of the interventions discussed have focused on one aspect of school aggression. Which of these approaches is the one to apply? How does one decide? To answer these questions one has to consider several factors, including the nature of the aggressive behavior, the student, and the context of the aggression. Simple, unilateral solutions are unlikely to ameliorate the complex of behaviors that are linked to school violence and vandalism.

AGGRESSION IN SCHOOL: MULTIPLE PERSPECTIVES

A multidimensional perspective toward school aggression involves various disciplines, theories, and interventions at different levels, goals, ideologies and values of all stakeholders or participants in the school. Teachers, parents, administrators, school boards, the community, and students all have a role. Also, the many facets of school aggression require an understanding of both its antecedents and consequences.

A violent and disruptive incident may be thought of as the concluding event in a chain of events leading to it. But several alternative hypothetical chains may be linked together for any specific act. In Figure 8.1, four such causal chains are proposed, each suggesting not only a different attribution for the violent act, but each also indicating different targets or levels of intervention within each chain. The problem can be conceptualized at an even more complex level when each of the four depicted chains is thought of as part of some larger system of linkages. What follows is an attempt to bring together the different, but overlapping, conceptual approaches to understanding the problem of aggressive school behavior. Each of these depictions is an attempt at a proposed solution to school violence or vandalism by providing a matrix through which the different dimensions of the problem are brought into focus; in sum, where the behavior, person, and environment can be viewed simultaneously.

In Table 8.1, the major dimensions are conceptualized in terms of both the goal of the intervention and the level at which it is implemented. The meaning of level — student, teacher, school, commun-

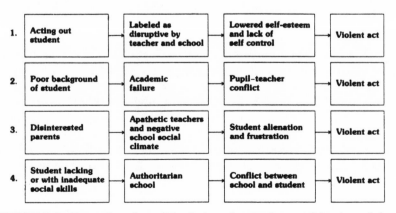

FIGURE 8.1. Examples of possible chains of causation resulting in a violent act. From Harootunian (1986, p. 131). Copyright 1986 Pergamon Press, Inc. Reprinted by permission.

TABLE 8.1. A Multilevel, Multigoal Solution Approach to School Violence

Level of intervention	Goal of intervention		
	Prevention	Compensatory	Remediation
Community	Adopt-a-school	Less restrictive child labor laws	Family support services Short-term treatment centers
School	24-hour custodial service	Use of plexiglass windows	Prescriptively tailored courses
Teacher	Programs to enhance knowledge of ethnic and minority milieu	Better teacher–pupil ratio	Acquisition of new training techniques in psychological skills, e.g., structured learning
Student	Identification cards	School transfers Part-time programs	Interpersonal training Behavior modification

Note. From Harootunian (1986, p. 131). Copyright 1986 Pergamon Press, Inc. Reprinted by permission.

ity—is clear. The intervention may focus on the aggressive student, provide the teacher with new knowledge, require changes in the curriculum, or initiate a program where various groups and businesses in the community "adopt a school." What may not be apparent from Table 8.1 is the idea that an intervention at one level may be only a partial resolution of the problem.

Levels of intervention in Table 8.1 mean that when aggression occurs, a response may involve more than just the disruptive student. Clearly it may require something to happen that involves the teacher, the school, or even the larger community. An approach at several levels is more likely to bring about positive results.

The goal of the intervention in Table 8.1 needs some additional explanation. Various actions taken against aggression are initiated to prevent or discourage hostile acts directed against persons or school property. Such measures as 24-hour custodial service and better lighting are designed to prevent aggression. The use of plexiglass windows may not prevent aggressive acts, but it will certainly reduce the incidence of broken windows. Compensatory interventions do not in themselves change aggressive or disruptive students, but they do offset the consequences of their actions. Remedial interventions, on the other hand, are aimed at changing students, not simply providing them with ways of circumventing their aggressive acts. In Table 8.1, this remediation is exemplified as prescriptively tailored courses, which at the student level may be implemented by specific applications of behavior

modification or courses designed to teach the students the basic interpersonal social skills they lack.

The key in Table 8.1 and the tables that follow is not a specific
intervention at a specific level, but rather seeing or looking at the whole
table as a systematic or total approach to school aggression. The proposed solution can then be better understood both in its intent and
consequences.

Table 8.2 has the same levels of intervention as Table 8.1, but its
second dimension describes the modes of intervention: psychological,
educational, administrative, legal, and physical. The latter may occur
separately or simultaneously. Modes of intervention simply are a way
of classifying or understanding the nature of an approach that may be
applied to curb aggression. Each mode taps different resources, some
of which may be outside of the school. The examples listed in Table
8.2 are some of the interventions reported in the literature. It should
be noted that some of the interventions appearing in Table 8.1 are also
in Table 8.2. For example, in both tables "interpersonal training" appears at the student level and presciptively tailored courses is found
at the school level. While both interventions are aspects of remediation in Table 8.1. According to Table 8.2, the intervention, interpersonal skills training is categorized under "psychological" while
prescriptively tailored course sequences is listed under "educational."

Tables 8.1 and 8.2 can be put together according to the three dimensions they represent. We leave it to readers to combine the dimen-

TABLE 8.2. A Multidimensional Intervention Strategy for School Violence

Level of intervention	Mode of intervention				
	Psychological	Educational	Administrative	Legal	Physical
Community	Program for disturbed children	Prosocial TV programs	Adopt-a-school programs	Gun control legislation	Near school, mobile home vandalism watch
School	Use of skilled conflict negotiators	Prescriptively tailored course se- quences	Reduction of class size	Legal rights handbook	Lighting, painting, paving programs
Teacher	Aggression management training	Enhanced knowledge of student ethnic milieu	Good teacher– pupil ratio	Compensation for aggression related ex- penses	Personal alarm systems
Student	Interpersonal skills training	Moral education	School transferr	Use of security personnel	Student murals, graffiti boards

sions of level, goal, and mode of intervention by their own graphic representation.

A multidimensional approach to school violence and vandalism, at first glance, might suggest an unnecessarily complex response to the problem. However, as our brief review has indicated, any one strategy in isolation often has resulted in confusion, if not contradictory findings. A multiple perspective strategy makes it possible to determine where a suggested intervention or approach fits and how it may influence or be influenced by adjacent solutions. Also a comprehensive view of school aggression may reveal gaps and overloads in the system. There is evidence, for example (Zwier & Vaughan, 1984), that almost one-half of the literature on school vandalism focuses on the physical dimensions of schools — better lighting, building design, and so on. The attempt is to make the buildings vandal proof.

What Tables 8.1 and 8.2 suggest is that interventions or strategies for the resolution of problems must be thought of as parts of a mosaic that represents the total ecology of school aggression. The tables serve as heuristics for understanding the complexity of aggressive behavior in and toward school.

There is yet another multidimensional way of looking at school violence and vandalism, and it is presented in Table 8.3. This presents a somewhat different view. Table 8.3 includes a mix of some of the categories of the previous tables, but introduces a different dimension worthy of note: ideological orientation. Zwier and Vaughan (1984) view ideological orientation as an essential aspect of understanding and solving the problem of school aggression. They state that "we must remember that the identification of the cause of a social problem is tantamount to the discovery of its solution" (p. 270).

The assumptions underlying the conservative, liberal, and radical ideologies, as defined by Zwier and Vaughan (1984) reflect issues which have involved participants in American schools for a long time. What is important is the congruence between a particular solution and an ideology. Table 8.3 shows that conservatively oriented individuals are likely to favor or suggest solutions such as better lighting, alarm systems, and so on. If, as noted previously, almost half of the interventions are of this sort, conservative ideologies would seem to be the dominant ones when school aggression is under consideration. Of course, there are a few instances of curriculum change and attempts at more student involvement in decisions that reflect respectively liberal and radical ideologies.

The linkage between ideology and the various attempts of solving problems of school aggression can be seen by viewing the various intersections in Tables 8.1 and 8.2 and determining the ideological orien-

TABLE 8.3. The Relationship Between Ideological Orientation, Assumption Concerning the Cause of School Vandalism, and Type of Solution Offered

Ideological orientation and assumption of cause	Type of solution		
	Specific ◄—————————————————► Diffuse		
	Physical environment	School system	Community at large
Conservative Vandals are deviant. They must be caught and punished.	Protection of school and school grounds, employment of security officers and caretakers[a]	Encouragement and enforcement of school rules, use of contingency contracts	Involvement of community in anti-vandalism patrols and (parent) restitution programs, dependence on judicial system
Liberal The school system is malfunctioning. Vandals capitalize on this.	(Superficial) improvement of the design, appearance, and layout of the school grounds	Modifications in school climate, curriculum, and use of special conflict management programs[a]	Extension of recreational activities, use of school after hours for health and social services
Radical The school system is debilitating. Vandalism is a response of normal individuals to abnormal conditions.	Promotion of radical changes in the structure and appearance of the school, approval of policy to decrease the size of large schools, and maintain small schools	Provision of student involvement in decision-making process, adoption of changes in assessment procedures, and exploration of alternative schooling methods	Involvement of the whole community in school affairs, installment of community education programs, improvement of social situation in society at large[a]

Note. From Zwier and Vaughan (1984, p. 269). Copyright 1984 the American Education Research Association. Reprinted by permission.
[a]The solution considered most favorably by the particular ideological orientation.

tation likely in favor of the particular solution. For a specific solution to be feasible, the values it elicits must to some extent overlap with the values or ideologies of those who are asked to accept and participate in its implementation. The greater the degree of congruence or acceptance of values between the proposed course of action and those who must act, the greater the likelihood the espoused goals will be gained.

In sum, this section has identified four dimensions of interventions that play a role in the struggle against aggressive behavior: goals, levels, modes, and ideological orientations. These dimensions are dynamic, interact with one another, and need to be understood better. The priority implication for practice is to begin thinking about school aggression in terms other than single, short-term, simple solutions. In the next section, we offer several suggestions for the prevention, reduction, and replacement of school aggression. Any single suggestion, if implemented, is likely to result in some improvement, but an organized set of them might have a more lasting effect. Such a set of interventions may be organized by going across a row in Table 8.1, down a column in Table 8.2, or using various other combinations.

SOME FEASIBLE IDEAS FOR SCHOOLS

There are some key "truths" to be communicated about teaching troubled and troubling students. First, our current diagnostic strategies are inadequate for the task of programming for students. Diagnoses that merely place children are wasteful of precious professional time. Second, teaching children depends on high-level teacher skills, but such skills are unlikely to develop in schools unless in-service, feedback, and modeling support are available to all the teachers. Third, the results of years of classroom research must be made available to both preservice and in-service teachers. To implement these findings, however, will often demand a restructuring of school schedules, professional relationships, and staffing patterns.

In-service training must be reconceptualized in many districts. Instead of the cafeteria style of training employed by many staff developers (e.g., workshops on "trendy" approaches, one-shot efforts with no follow-up), systematic approaches with long-term goals and evaluation must be employed. Teachers learn the way students learn. Their training experiences should be as carefully planned as the students' academic year goals are developed.

Building-level support must be in place to gain and maintain skills. Just as children learn best with continuous feedback, so too, teachers will improve when there are many opportunities for observation and feedback. Much of this feedback should be considered formative evaluation. Teachers should not be penalized for not knowing a skill. Poor evaluations should be based on unwillingness to learn and/or experiment with strategies that are known to be effective in improving achievement and behavior.

Students achieve at different rates. Some in-class programs are possible. Social skills training (McGinnis & Goldstein, 1984) is an important building block for any instructional program. Classroom meetings that teach impulse control and problem solving are critical forums in schools within a democratic society.

Every school needs ongoing programs in parent education, children-of-divorce groups, individual psychotherapy, and case management. These are not frills in today's world. They are tied directly to student's abilities to profit from educational interventions (Swap, 1987).

The development of such programs will depend on a highly motivated and cooperative staff. Administrators must value such activities so that teachers, psychologists, and other specialists are not unintentionally penalized for their commitment to children.

What follows are some more specific recommendations to counter school violence and vandalism. Each of these suggestions needs to viewed tentatively and not as the solution to the problem by itself. As Feldhusen (1979) has noted, we may know the problem of aggression very well, its causes moderately well, and its solutions least well. On the basis of the current state of knowledge, the following recommendations seem warranted as ways of reducing school aggression:

- Positive behavior of students should be rewarded and recognized much more than it is now.
- The principal should have discretionary resources available and must take the initiative in creating a positive humanistic climate in the school.
- All constituencies of the school—teachers, students, administrators, and parents—should cooperate in the development and enforcement of school rules.
- Special courses and other explicit efforts must be made to help students develop self-control, self-direction, conflict resolution, and personal management.
- Multiple measures of success in school should be utilized. Grades should not be the sole measure of success.
- Illegal behavior in the school should not be condoned. Crime and delinquency should be prosecuted.
- Schools should offer alternative programs that meet the individual needs of noncollege-bound youngsters.
- In-service programs such as teaching techniques of behavior management should be developed for teachers and administrators.
- Task forces and other linkages should be established between and among parents, administrators, teachers, and students to assess and develop plans for combating school crime.
- Counseling services for the family, and for family and school staff together should be available to resolve conflicts among parents, students, and school personnel.
- School should have a coordinated guidance system to diagnose, plan, and assess programs for disruptive students.
- Teachers should have clear and explicit objectives and standards, particularly when teaching skills that are prerequisites to further learning.

- Work-study and career education programs should be available for students.
- School buildings should be used during the evenings and weekends to serve the community.
- Teachers and administrators should live in the community.
- Security guards and devices should be employed to protect students and staff from perpetrators of violence from both inside and outside of schools that have severe problems.
- For students with serious behavior problems, special settings should be created for short-term treatment.

Which, if any, of these recommendations will be appropriate in a specific school will depend, of course, on the circumstances. We offer these recommendations not as simple prescriptions but as some apparently viable steps that can be taken to curb school crime. Public schools in America a tremendous array of tasks, and some say this has brought "purposive disorder" into the school (Sennett, 1980). But when the "purposive disorder" has been accompanied by increases in violence, vandalism, theft, arson, and so on, it is time for the school to consider some of the alternatives we have just presented. Curbing school crime will require more than the everyday response, as indicated by the following quotation:

It seems to be characteristic of the creation of settings (although by no means peculiar to it) that there is no systematic effort to understand the universe of alternatives of thought and action relevant to any decision that has to be made. For any step in the growth of the setting, there is always a universe of alternatives which could be considered, but in practice there seems to be awareness only of a very constricted universe, and this is largely due to the weight of tradition, a pessimistic assessment of what others will allow, and the lack of an organizational vehicle devoted to a description of the universe of alternatives. The results are that virtues are made of presumed necessities, courage is not seen as a relevant characteristic, and imagination is viewed as a luxury relevant to some future world and not the present one. When the concept of the universe and alternatives is taken seriously, the personal consequences can be as profound as the intellectual ones. (Sarason, Zitnay, & Grossman, 1971, pp. 91–92)

Although there is no simple panacea to school violence, it has been and can be confronted successfully by schools and school personnel who have been creative risk takers. Throughout, the underlying theme has been that the reduction of school violence will require a renewed spirit of cooperation and effort on the part of all of the constituencies encompassing the school. Not one of the just-cited recommendations can be implemented without consideration of some of the others. If, for example, formal mechanisms are established for student participation in the governance of the school, the students may relegate this responsibility to teachers and administrators, not because they are indifferent to the school, but because they have never adequately mastered the necessary basic social and political skills that will enable them to participate. Providing instruction in these basic skills may, in turn, require teachers to participate in in-service education to acquire the requisite knowledge and skills. Thus, a chain of events is precipitated which can be understood through the ecological perspective of the school, a perspective which promises payoff in combating school violence.

Sarason (1982) has essentially detailed a similar approach. He has analyzed the problem of changing the school from various perspectives. One implication of his analysis is that the aspect or part of the school one deals with affects how it is seen in relationship to the whole as well as the other parts. This perception influences such consequences as the definition of the school's problems, their priorities, their solutions, and so forth.

The thesis of this chapter from the start has been that many of the research findings and intervention attempts regarding school aggression have emphasized the "parts" at the expense of the "whole." If future such endeavors are to pay off, it would appear that strategies based on the "whole" will be more productive—strategies such as those laid out in this chapter.

CHAPTER 9

✛

The Family

There is overwhelming evidence that many children and youth who engage in serious aggressive behaviors have experienced some disruption in their own families or communities. These young people may be the offspring of antisocial parents (Farrington, 1987; Frick, Lahey, Loeber, & Stouthamer-Loeber, 1992; Robins & Earls, 1985; Robins & Ratcliff, 1979) or have been raised in homes or neighborhoods plagued by poverty, drug abuse, domestic violence, disorganization, or racism (Elliott, Huizinga, & Ageton, 1985; Rutter & Giller, 1983; Wilson & Herrnstein, 1985). Families that are characterized by harsh and inconsistent discipline, little positive parent involvement, and poor supervision are at greatest risk of having antisocial children (Loeber & Dishion, 1983; McCord, McCord, & Howard, 1963; Patterson, DeBaryshe, & Ramsey, 1989). To maximize the effectiveness of any treatment plan for aggressive youth, a cooperative or concurrent intervention with family is critical.

Analogous to suggestions given earlier, interventions that offer new skills to young people and simultaneously change their environments are the most likely to succeed. In the best of situations, schools and families would join together to assist troubled youth, and in so doing evaluate their own policies, procedures, beliefs, and expectations as these interact with goals to reduce aggression and increase security in school and in homes.

Successful treatment most certainly depends on strategies that involve school, home, and community. This view is based on available research (e.g., Lewis, 1982; Jones, Weinrott, & Howard, 1981) and on an ecological theory of human behavior.

Before describing ways to enhance home–school collaboration and multisystem programs, the following section will outline the basic tenets of ecological theory. Ecological theory can provide a framework within which to plan and evaluate prevention efforts and treatment for individuals, classroom, families, and communities. It is a helpful conceptual and practical tool.

ECOLOGICAL THEORY

Proponents of the ecological orientation take the position that behavior is determined by the *interaction* of individual and environmental characteristics. Although all major approaches to understanding human behavior cite internal and external forces as operating together to produce behavior, they differ significantly in emphasis.

For example, both psychodynamic and biophysical models are concerned for the most part with the definition and understanding of internal forces. Psychodynamic theorists focus primarily on "needs" and "drives" and on the investigation of patterns of behavior that occur at various stages of development. Biophysical theorists, on the other hand, emphasize physiological conditions or gene interactions that may lead to certain typical behavior patterns.

Behavioral and sociological models are concerned mainly with external forces. The behavior theorist tries to understand stimulus–response patterns and the reinforcing and punishing conditions in the environment that produce particular sequences of behaviors. This is a functional analysis of behavior. Sociologists are more concerned with the broader environment including institutions, communities, culture, and society in their efforts to understand conditions that produce individual and group behavior.

Ecological theory maintains an equal emphasis on internal and external forces when attempting to understand human behavior; ecologists assume there is a unique pattern of explanatory forces for each individual case under scrutiny. Gordon (1982), describing ecological theory, has noted:

> While the individual is being examined, the model simultaneously permits the worker to study the environment, seeking beneficial changes in the total structure, redefining the goals, and exploring the ability of the client to survive in that state, as well as the potential of both for changed existence in improved states. (p. 110)

Examine Figure 9.1 as a depiction of the relationship of ecological theory to other models of understanding human behavior, especially troubled human behavior.

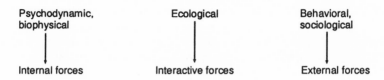

FIGURE 9.1. Conceptualizations of human behavior.

Ecologists examine ecosystems rather than individuals. Ecosystems are composed of all the interacting systems of living things and their nonliving surroundings. Ecosystems have histories and internal development that make each unique and constantly changing. When a child appears "normal," ecologists see the ecosystem as congruent or balanced. On the other hand, when such congruence does not exist, the child is likely to be considered deviant (i.e., out of harmony with social norms) or incompetent (i.e., unable to perform purposefully in the unchanged setting). When this is the case, ecologists say the system is not balanced, that particular elements are in conflict with one another. Such conflicts are termed "points of discordance," that is, specific places where there is a failure to match between the child and his or her ecosystem.

Historical Antecedents

Ecology is not seen usually as a separate discipline, but rather as an area of study within several disciplines. Basic concepts have come from a variety of fields other than psychology, for example, education, biology, sociology, and anthropology. Despite the diversity of disciplines represented, scientists interested in ecology are always concerned about the relationship of individuals to settings and use similar research methods in their inquiries. All human ecologists would agree that behavior is a product of the interaction between internal forces and the environmental circumstances.

Anthropologists may have been the original human ecologists. Their contributions to an understanding of troubled or psychopathological behavior have focused primarily on the cultural contexts in which deviant behavior occurs. Sociologists have added to the knowledge base in human ecology with studies of the significant social conditions that tend to be associated with high rates of deviance. Farris and Dunham (1939), in their classic work *Mental Disorders in Urban Areas,* described their conceptions of "concentric zone theory" and social disorganization, and the relationship of those concepts to mental illness. They proposed three things as necessary to have a mentally healthy child: a) intimacy and affection between the child and some permanent group; b) a consistency of influence; and c) some harmony between home and outside situations. Each of their criteria is an interactive one. They also noted that "insanity" is not defined by a list of actions but, rather, by a lack of fit between actions and situations.

Some of the earliest and most important applications of ecological theory to the treatment of special needs children were done by William Rhodes. In 1967 he suggested that special educators had borrowed a biophysical model and attempted to apply it to troubled children. As a result, educators had come to view disturbance as residing totally and completely within the child, and consequently their intervention efforts were based on finding and correcting the neurological, chemical, genetic, and/or psychological flaws within youngsters. Rhodes proposed an alternative view of emotional disturbance that emphasized the reciprocal nature of disturbance and focused on the interchange between a child and the surrounding environment. Although not denying influence from other sources, Rhodes contended that at the very least, both the child and the environment were likely intervention targets. The goals and assumptions of ecological theory in treating troubled children have been further developed by Apter (1977, 1982), Hobbs (1966, 1975), Kounin (1970, 1975), and Swap (1974, 1978).

Ecological psychologists (e.g. Barker, 1978; Lewin, 1951) have analyzed settings in terms of both psychological and nonpsychological forces. Barker and his colleagues developed a comprehensive research program designed to operationalize the concept of "life space" developed by Kurt Lewin. In their work on behavior settings (small ecosystems that call forth particular behaviors), they have discovered the importance of "synomorphy"—the fit of individual behavior to the particular setting—and concluded, as did Farris and Dunham (1939), that mental illness is a term used to represent behavior that is poorly fitted to the setting.

Medical ecologists have also contributed to an understanding of human behavior through research into the interaction between individual genetic determinants and environmental differences (Buss & Plomin, 1984; Plomin, 1989; Plomin, Pedersen, McClearn, Nesselroade, & Bergeman, 1988). Thomas, Chess, and Birch (1968) found that infants are born with varying levels of nine temperamental dimensions (i.e., activity level, approach/withdrawal, intensity of reaction, quality of mood, attention span and persistence, rhythmicity, adaptability, threshold of responsiveness, and distractibility). They suggested that any level of these qualities, more recently referred to as EAS (emotionality, activity, sociability) can result in emotional disturbance under cer-

tain environmental conditions, that is, the temperaments (and consequently the behavior) of some children fit better into their environments than do the temperaments and behaviors of other's.

Critical Elements of Ecological Theory

1. *Each child is an inseparable part of a small social system.* Every child
lives in a context that is both unique and critical to our understanding
of the youngster and our intervention efforts.

2. *Disturbance is viewed not as a disease located within the body of the
child but, rather, as discordance in the system.* Contrary to psychodynamic
or biophysical models in which the disease defined the child, from the
ecological position the troubled youngster represents a troubled system. For example, environments may elicit disturbing behaviors and
then identify and label such behaviors as symptoms of emotional disturbance or behavior disorder. Which behaviors get labeled depends
upon the time, place, and culture in which they are emitted and upon
the tolerance of those who observe them (Swap, Prieto, & Harth, 1982;
Rhodes, 1967). This view does not negate the role played by genetics
but acknowledges that genetic effects on behavior are polygenetic and
probabilistic.

3. *Discordance may be defined as a disparity between an individual's abilities and the demands or expectations of the environment—a failure to match
between child and system.* Some settings are extremely demanding and unresponsive to the individual abilities of a child. In such environments,
a child may appear incompetent while in other, more nurturing environments, the same child will not be identified as deviant. An example may be the so-called "six-hour retarded child"—a child labeled as
retarded by the school but considered normal in the family and community.

Goals and Purposes

In sum, the goal of an ecologically based intervention is not a particular state of mental health or set of behavior patterns, but rather an increased concordance between the behavior of a child and the settings
in which he or she resides. These goals are reached by using existing
techniques in an ecological manner. The treatment plan is guided by
the child interacting with all the important elements of his or her life
space. The ecological perspective is a useful umbrella to organize a variety of intervention efforts into a purposeful attempt to increase the

possibility of system change, the competence of individuals, and the congruence of individuals with their settings.

APPLICATIONS TO INTERVENTION

With ecological concepts as a backdrop, what services beyond the school are most likely to be useful to children and youth who engage in aggressive behaviors? Clearly, a synthesis among family, medical, mental health, educational, social service, and legal–judicial systems is called for to ensure that unique needs of young people receive appropriate attention.

Any service must, of course, meet certain criteria to improve the probabilities of success. Change is most often needed if successful programming is to occur in the following respects:

1. *More effective use of resources.* The tremendous number of youngsters with continuing skill deficits and unmet emotional needs, in spite of the conglomerate of efforts by all systems, demands that existing resources be used more effectively. In mental health, this may be seen in a variety of efforts to develop programs that will lead to the prevention of emotional disturbances by reorganizing the way in which professionals spend their time. As an example, Caplan (1970) provided a model of consultation that has changed the nature of many psychiatrists' and psychologists' work from one-to-one efforts with patients to consultation with others who work with those clients. A consultation model can help spread the effects of professional expertise by enabling a single professional to reach many more troubled people through the appropriate sharing of his or her knowledge and skills.

Simply stated, although new services are always welcome, a very real problem is the poor utilization or deployment of existing services.

2. *Better communication.* Although the "communication problem" has become a cliché in modern times, it is no less real in relationships between the systems mentioned above than in the families of troubled children. As Unger (1974) has noted about the social welfare system,

> It should be clear that a lack of communication within the social welfare bureaucracy and between the system and other suppliers of services (agencies, groups, individuals) is a problem which creates many other problems. But what is not clear from the above is that communication between the system and the client is also frequently poor. The client may wait for months for a much needed service and not once hear from a worker that something is being done and that he has not been simply forgotten or ignored. (p. 398)

It is imperative that systems find ways of overcoming the rigidity that always develops in small or large bureaucracies and begin responding to the real needs of clients. Children and families need information about available services, and if communication is to improve, such data probably must come from a single and credible source. More and more programs and agencies are using the role of advocate or coordinator or primary worker as an effective way to build a partnership between clients and programs.

3. *Better recognition of historical impact.* The ways in which we provide services to troubled children today are greatly influenced by practices and programs of earlier times. The lasting effect of buildings is especially powerful, as Rhodes and Gibbins (1972) have noted:

> Any social institutional form that includes buildings and facilities has a tenacious capacity for maintaining itself within the social body. These edifices have a powerful influence on the way in which communities continue to handle human problems no matter what new discoveries or methods may evolve.... Society seems very reluctant to fully abandon either a frame of reference or a facility that it has brought into existence to handle a human problem. Most characteristically, the new dominating frame of reference is imposed on the old one, like a new archaeological layer on an older deposit. (p. 362)

Historically, intervention efforts have focused on correcting the deficits(s) in the disturbed child. This strategy of intervention may have come about because: (a) disturbed children threaten the community and require a corrective response (Rhodes, 1967); (b) the dominance of the medical model made such individual treatment the logical response; or, (c) political action is taken to remedy the problems presented by the individuals. Whatever the reasons, professionals at work in the systems we have been discussing must be cautious of the effects of history on their settings and programs and roles.

Having outlined some hallmarks of effective service and the issues to monitor while planning and implementing services, the subsequent sections of this chapter will explore service options that capture the spirit of ecological theory. These services are aimed primarily at families.

HOME-SCHOOL COLLABORATION

Guidelines for improving the partnership between families and schools follow. These suggestions have been useful for many schools with many different types of families. No illusion if offered, however, in terms of the ease with which many parents of aggressive young people can be involved with the schools. These families are often the "tough" ones to connect with. Early and persistent efforts are absolutely necessary. It may also be necessary to look into the child's life to identify an available adult—grandparent, aunt or uncle, older sibling, and so on. Further, parents of well-adjusted children can play an important role in supporting safe environments for all young people if these parents can be mobilized.

Apart from offering services to problem children, what other modifications might schools make that would be responsive to families? A school interested in supporting the adjustment of families who are dealilng with an aggressive child might consider changes in information transfer, intensity of shared involvement, interaction and shared responsibility, and decision making. In addition, early identification of vulnerable youth and families is critical.

Information Transfer

Information provision and sharing is a type of joining with parents. Traditionally, this has meant providing parents with report cards, notes, or phone calls in addition to infrequent parent teacher meetings. It has also involved getting fairly superficial information from parents about their children. To make this a meaningful exchange, several things could happen at a school (Alexander, Kroth, Simpson, & Poppelreiter, 1982; Conoley, 1987; Ehly, Conoley, & Rosenthal, 1985; Hughes & Baker, 1990; Lombard, 1979; Losen & Diament, 1978; Loven, 1978):

Forms

Because a disproportionate number of aggressive youths come from divorced or separated families, forms that collect information about families should include queries about the address, phone number, and involvement of noncustodial parents. Some noncustodial parents are prevented by court order from interacting with their children, but most would benefit from being on school mailing lists to receive notices of activities. School personnel must ensure that noncustodial parents are permitted contact with their children (restraining orders may be most common in families racked by violence) so these parents can be helpful backups for the custodial parent.

In addition, such forms might routinely ask parents about the young person's favorite reinforcers, what situations at home are predictably troublesome to handle, and what the parents' typical discipline plan entails. Although the use of such information may be only indirect, school officials can begin a process in kindergarten of seeking parental input and asking about important family challenges.

Communication Skills

Teachers and administrators can be trained in appropriate communication skills that emphasize conflict resolution, mediation, and responses to angry confrontations. These skills may be useful with both the young people and their families.

Content Information about Aggression

Teachers can receive specialized training about holding parent–teacher meetings and other forms of parent communication with a special focus on the stresses and strains of parenting aggressive youth. Teachers should know about coercive communication patterns (Bramblett, Wodarski, & Thyer, 1991; Patterson, 1982; Snyder, 1977; Snyder & Patterson, 1986) and be able to provide helpful suggestions to break these negative cycles between parents and their children. Teachers should receive regular updates from their administrators about security programs that are underway in their schools so that such information can be shared with anxious parents.

Parental Expertise

Parents must be seen and responded to as experts on their own children and as such be asked to provide the school with continuous feedback on the status of their children. For example, parents might be encouraged to keep the school informed about legal activities that involve the children, traumatic incidents a child might have witnessed, and so on. This information may be very useful for school personnel in interpreting child behavior and may assist parents and children by focusing attention on children's experiences of coming to schools where violence is a daily occurrence.

Communication Alternatives

Every school should have a regular means of communicating with parents, for example, through the use of newsletters, phone committees, community bulletin boards, features in newspapers, and monthly meetings. School bulletins could highlight especially appropriate TV, movie, or book resources for parents to use with their children. A variety of methods may be especially helpful in one- parent homes. Often the work schedules of single parents make regular attendance at school functions very difficult.

Case Manager

A coordinator of information and services should be available to every parent, so the parent has one person to contact to help through the school bureaucracy. Noncustodial parents may be especially helped by the existence of a "case-manager" role because their information about their children may be incomplete. Coordinating special services for young people is a far more vital role than often imagined, and part of that challenge is keeping everyone informed.

Reading Materials

Specialized bibliographies and reading materials should be made available to parents, depending on their particular needs. These would be useful in the school library, but equally helpful if disseminated to parents.

Parents might also be given very practical lists of suggestions regarding child safety. Almost twenty years ago the Parents' Network of the National Committee for Citizen in Education (NCCE) produced a list of do's and don'ts that is still quite applicable.

Don't
- Send your child to school early without being sure another adult on the school end knows about it and approves.
- Ignore your children if they complain or say they are worried about being in certain places in the school or on the school grounds.
- Allow your children to remain in or around school buildings after school is over. If you pick them up and can't get there at the regular time, advise your children and make arrangements with someone you trust to pick them up for you.
- Assume that the present security system for the school is the best possible. Ask about how visitors are handled—how access to doors is controlled. Ask for written information on these matters, review it, think about it, and ask questions. Make suggestions.
- Try to correct the problems in your school on your own. The odds are very high against success if you go it alone. Get others to join you.

Do
- Caution your children about talking with adults they don't recognize while in school in the halls, bathrooms or other places.

- Talk with school personnel about using children to run errands. This usually means they would be alone and increases danger to their safety.
- Encourage your child to report trouble — lunch money taken, physically roughed up, threatened. There seems to be plenty of convincing evidence that part of the reason things have reached the crisis stage is that more and more people (adults and other students) began to realize that there was only a slim chance anyone would report the problem. If you do this, please remember the children deserve protection if someone tries to get back at them; assure them something will be done to follow-up on their report.
- Encourage your junior and senior high age child to think about talking with their friends if they are worried about violence in their schools and seeing if they want to form their own committee or become a part of a larger committee which includes adults.
- Make sure the rules, regulations and expectations you have for your child are clearly understood and followed. Remember your attitude is bound to set a tone for school behavior and response to school rules. (NCCE, 1975, pp. 21–22)

Parental Visits

Parents should routinely be invited to speak to children in their areas of expertise. This should happen frequently. Programs that emphasize parental contributions link parents to everyday learning objectives for children and can increase parents' investment in the schooling process.

In addition, the mere presence of parents (especially fathers) has been found in some school districts to reduce the occurrence of violence. A few schools have reported organizing "security dads" to attend pep rallies and dances. A school thinking of doing this should plan to offer some training, as fathers may not necessarily understand mediation and conflict resolution.

Intense Collaboration

Another aspect of partnership involves collaborative home–school programs that might include, for example, instructions for tutoring a child, teaching prosocial skills, or implementation of solutions or rewards.

Although most families can benefit from this kind of collaboration with teachers and other school professionals, families struggling with delinquent youth are in great need of adult support. A most common concern of parents is the lack of other supportive adults with whom to solve problems. When families have a history of involvement with the judicial–legal system, they can become distrustful of outsiders and fail to develop supportive social networks.

Hallmarks of successful collaborative efforts are as follows:

1. *All parties must understand exactly the changes expected of each.* Everyone—teacher, parent, and child—must agree to a change. Already overwhelmed parents cannot be asked to make dramatic changes in their typical coping styles. Some sensitive approaches that rely on small adjustments, coupled with support, are necessary.

2. *A feasible communication system between parents and teachers must be established.* Parents can be difficult to contact. Often it is useful to have alternative contacts such as childcare workers or grandparents.

3. *Consistent follow-through on the parts of teachers and parents in terms of their behaviors and any rewards that have been agreed upon must be facilitated.* Professionals attempting a collaborative program may need to allot more time than usual to support the parents in making changes. Parents' own agendas and potential deficits in parenting skills can interfere with follow-through on behavioral contracts.

Often, cooperative effort is aimed at fairly discrete child behaviors (e.g., amount of homework being turned in, spelling scores, off-task behavior), but can be the vehicle for classroom and family change if all parties live up to their contracts. For example, parents who follow through with positive attention to a child who performs well at school are likely to improve not only the child's school work, but also the parent–child relationship. Analogously, a teacher who communicates frequently with parents is likely to be more successful with individual children and to feel more supported by parents in doing difficult work.

Interaction and Shared Responsibility

The active involvement of parents at the school represents an important way to enhance home–school collaboration. Unfortunately, most American families no longer include a parent who is routinely available for school duties. Lightfoot (1978) emphasizes the importance of such interaction, however:

> Not only does the working collaboration of parents and teachers transform the educational environment and cultural medium of the school, it also changes the adult perceptions of their roles and relationships. (p. 173)

Volunteer Programs

Lightfoot goes on to say that school volunteer mothers reported that many behavioral and learning problems in school disappeared when their children experienced an alliance between mothers and teachers. In addition, they were able to share important information with teachers about neighborhood children; they reduced the workload of teachers; they gained an appreciation of how complex and burdensome teaching is, and finally, they began to perceive the school as belonging to them. These outcomes have been replicated in several inner-city schools (Comer, 1984, 1987; Comer & Haynes, 1991; Lightfoot, 1976).

To make a volunteer program work with families, everyone will have to agree that it is important. Mothers and fathers must be trained in diverse roles (Cowen et al., 1975); childcare must be engineered for nonschool aged children; some kind of real reward or motivational system must be in place for volunteers; teachers must be convinced and then trained to use help effectively; and, someone must be in charge of coordination.

In addition, volunteers must be organized with parents' limited time taken into account. For example, over the course of an academic year parents might be asked to help with one field trip, bake cookies for one party, read stories in the library for only one 30-minute period, or supervise the crosswalk on only one morning. Although this kind of program involves complex organization, the payoffs could be significant.

Childcare

Many American families have difficulty arranging for high quality daycare for their children. Many schools now offer early morning programs and care until about five o'clock. These programs, although not evaluated to our knowledge, seem to offer parents peace of mind and children a significantly safer environment that that of an empty house.

Childcare should also be made available during parent–teacher conferences and school plays or concerts. Often such care is free, but even a nominal charge might be acceptable to parents. If every parent paid only a dollar for an hour of care, junior or senior high students could still receive attractive pay for entertaining a group of children. If parents know they can attend functions without finding care for their other children *and* can look forward to an enjoyable time, their participation might increase in the lives of school-aged children.

Finally, Swap (1992) reported on a school facilitating a partnership among the school, parents, and local businesses to arrange for care for mildly ill children. The model she presented illustrates a home-based approach for children who were between 9 and 12. Visiting nurses stopped in and checked on children during their sick days. Other possibilities include shared sponsorship of centers that care for children with colds, ear infections, and other fairly routine illnesses.

Such programs are established with joint funding from parents and local private industry. The businesses have often been approached and influenced by school personnel who solicit contributions based on family needs and on the benefits to industry from decreased worker absenteeism.

Although no link has been established between aggression and being sick, a link has been found between supervision and delinquent behavior in males (Loeber & Dishion, 1983). Any programs that organize increased supervision and monitoring of children is a preventive effort toward reducing externalizing behaviors.

Decision Making

Ultimately, children and families are assisted through difficult situations by receiving support to get on with their lives in prosocial ways. The exact path for any particular family toward this goal will be impossible for school personnel to recognize without input from parents. In like manner, parents have difficulty making the best decisions because of the emotionality that can surround parenting a child who seems out of control. However, in real partnership with each other, professionals and parents might assist children in important ways. Some suggestions follow.

First, schools can sponsor parent training workshops that are based on needs actually identified by parents. These workshops may be about learning games, nutritional snacks, or prosocial communication. Bringing people together in problem-solving groups increases their abilities to deal with stress (Pilisuk, 1982). A study by Lindblad-Goldberg and Dukes (1985) suggested that more adaptive mothers had more nonfamily support than less adaptive mothers. Family members, mentioned often by both groups, provided support, but also made intense demands upon the mothers. Schools, never mentioned as supportive by either group—despite the fact that both groups were receiving services from a clinic because of their children's problems in school—could be a wellspring of such nonfamily support.

Second, the school building can be used as a community center where adult education classes are taught, children play sports, senior citizens meet, and local law enforcement officials teach about safety

and crime prevention. Creating a community center for families search-
ing for safe places for their children may be a very important contribution. The center must be safe, however, necessitating close cooperation with community leaders and police.

This suggestion falls short of programs that are actually community schools. Although evaluation of community-run schools is positive
with regard to acts of vandalism, differences among schools called "community schools" make clear directives difficult to discern.

Third, school buses could be made available to carry mothers or
fathers and their school children to libraries, museums, or special ex-
hibits. The economic stress experienced by many families can limit their
activities and their energy to organize events with their children. This
unfortunate reality contributes to unstructured and unsupervised time
for children. Such times are an invitation for children to victimize
others or be victimized.

Finally, brief family consultations or counseling could become an
integral part of educational programming for children. Application of
work coming from the Oregon Social Learning Center by Patterson
and his associates may serve as a useful basis for this mode of service (Fogatch, Patterson, & Skinner, 1990; Patterson, 1982; Patterson,
1986; Patterson & Dishion, 1988; Patterson, Reid, Jones, & Conger,
1975).

Parents of antisocial children have often been found to reinforce
coercive cycles of communication and behavior in the home. These
cycles escalate over time resulting in increasingly serious aggressive
events. Parents of these children have been seen to be noncontingent
toward both prosocial and aggressive behavior from their children.
They may laugh at or attend to inappropriate behavior many times each
day while ignoring prosocial behaviors. Further, children of these
families often use coercive, negative behaviors to escape interactions
with other members of the family. In this way, the coercive behaviors
are both rewarded, and are somewhat functional, in highly aversive environments.

Treatment based on this conceptualization highlights training the
parents to change their communication patterns and the discipline
methods that characterize their families. They also learn to increase
the supervision of their children. Treatment has been most successful
with younger children (Kazdin, 1987) and should be combined with
social skills training and academic remediation to increase the probabilities of success (Patterson, DeBaryshe, & Ramsey, 1989).

The critical point to make here is that parents and school professionals must come together to identify concerns and solutions; shared
decision making increases investment (Lundquist, 1982).

Summary

For at least 10 years we have known that in most cases the exact treat-ment offered to troubled and troubling children and youths is less im-portant than the coordination of the systems interacting with the child. This becomes most evident when children are discharged from residen-tial treatment facilities. Their progress within the facility and the type of treatment offered to them are only minimally correlated with out-comes (health, vocation, education, etc.). The best predictor of good outcome is a harmonized receiving system — the family is prepared, the school has developed a plan, there is outpatient followup, and com-munity resources are in place (Lewis, 1982). It follows that in develop-ing a treatment model we should use what we know creates positive long-term outcomes for children and youth.

Recall Farris and Dunham's (1939) idea that to enjoy mental health a child requires (a) intimacy and affection between the child and some permanent group, (b) a consistency of influence, and (c) some harmo-ny between home and outside situations. Although these concepts are abstract, they can be used to judge any program that is offered. For example, has a stable and loving environment been established for a child? Are the people in that environment trained to exert a consis-tent positive influence on the child? Does that environment have clear and helpful liaisons with all the other systems that affect the child? When these questions are answered in the affirmative, the child is positioned for normal development.

For these reasons, collaboration between schools and families is vital for positive outcomes with young people. These two institutions have the potential to create intimacy and affection with a child and a consistent positive influence. School personnel cannot rely on every family, but they can revise their procedures and policies to bring as many families into partnership as possible.

Consider Figure 9.2 as a summary model of home–school collabor-ation. Good schools with teachers who are excellent instructors have the potential to enhance both child and family functioning. We know that when children are more involved in their schools — suggesting that schools be organized in ways to facilitate many forms of involvement — rates of behavior disorder are low (Barker, 1968; Barker & Gump, 1964; Boyer, 1983; Glass, Cahen, Smith, & Filby, 1982; Goodlad, 1984, Plath, 1965; Sizer, 1984). Schools that pay attention to the stresses of transi-tions (e.g., from elementary to junior high school) are more successful in keeping dropout rates low (Felner, Ginter, & Primavera, 1982; Sim-mons, Burgeson, Carlton-Ford, & Blyth, 1987). Attention to teaching behaviors and indicators of school effectiveness are vital to enhance

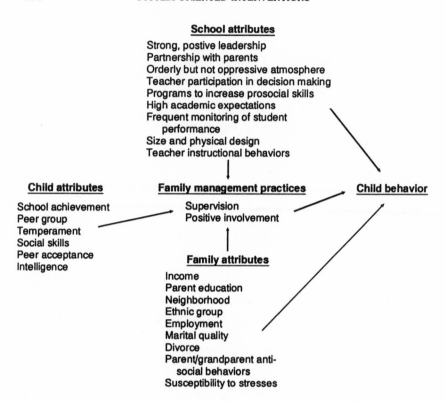

FIGURE 9.2. School and family attributes relating to child outcomes.

a school's chance to influence children and families (Brophy, 1986; Patterson et al., 1989; Good & Weinstein, 1986; Purkey & Smith, 1983; Rutter, 1983).

Other aspects of the model focus on child temperament, the skills of the parents, and the situation of the family in terms of socioeconomic level. Only continued research will verify the role played by each variable that is mentioned. This graphic helps us understand the child's world as one that is transactional/ecological. Attention must be directed to the patterns of social relations, connections, or linkages in every setting inhabited by young people (Linney & Seidman, 1989; Seidman, 1988).

INTERVENTION OUTSIDE THE FAMILY

Although the purview of this chapter is primarily the family, additional information about community treatment options for aggressive youth is also important to consider. These include residential treatment for youth and community programs.

Residential Treatment

Unfortunately, there is limited information about effective treatments outside of families and schools. Inpatient care, day treatment or partial hospitalization, group homes, individual outpatient treatment, respite services, wilderness therapy, and therapeutic foster care have all been modes of service delivery for troubled and troubling youth.

Most of the time, aggressive adolescent males, especially those who exhibited antisocial behavior in late childhood or early adolescence, are quite resistant to treatment (Farrington, 1983; Farrington, Gallagher, Morley, St. Ledger, & West, 1986; Loeber, 1982). Some research suggests that long-term care for this group in residential treatment facilities is promising (Colyar, 1991; Kazdin, 1987). The current cost of such treatment makes it an option for only the smallest minority of youngsters.

Many youngsters actually do quite well in their treatment facilities. The goal of treatment is, however, successful reintegration into the community. Although some short-term improvements are apparent after discharge, most of these disappear unless some significant changes have occurred in the family, school, and community's readiness to cope with the young person. This circle of influence is critical to success.

If parents are making a choice for an out-of-home placement, certain components should be investigated. For example, how extensive is the family therapy program? What extension services does the placement offer to the school following discharge? Will treatment be offered or is diagnosis the main goal of the hospitalization? Does the treatment reflect an emphasis on cognitive–behavioral goals? Are vocational, academic, social, and emotional objectives part of the treatment? What are the characteristics of the other clients? Does the facility match the problem? Particularly if the problem is behavioral, is the facility a residential treatment center in contrast to a hospital?

Although little research exists for determining the optimal components of out-of-home care, an ecological framework suggests the critical components of good care.

Beyond investigating the accreditation of a particular treatment facility and the credentials of the staff, most parents and educators have only limited knowledge of how to choose a residential program. It may be useful to consider the following:

Assessment

Assessments should be profile analyses, that is, the following questions should be answered:

- What are functional needs of children and youths?
- What are their strengths, their deficits?
- Where are the points of discordance?
- What are short- and long-term goals?
- What is the capacity of the current family and school systems to respond?
- What modifications must be made and what supports offered to family and school to match the young persons needs?
- Who will be responsible for the program?
- How will success be evaluated?

Assessment procedures must result in more than a diagnosis. Unlike many purely medical–biophysical testing, finding a psychological diagnosis rarely gives unequivocal direction for treatment. Although finding out what's wrong may seem important, the most challenging aspect of helping troubled youth is coming up with a plan the young person and all the related adults can carry out. Motivating and supporting others to follow through on treatment is the most difficult task of the therapist.

Treatments

Results of meta-analyses of child therapy (e.g., Casey & Berman, 1985; Tuma, 1990) give hope that psychological treatment makes a positive difference for children and youth. Cognitive–behavioral approaches, especially within the context of family intervention, may be the most powerful of the current technologies. Good residential or hospital programs should have social skills training, interpersonal problem-solving and decision-making training, vocational exploration and development, health and sexuality education, educational programs suitable for the grade level of the young person, family outreach, moral education, and aggression replacement therapy. Parents should be wary of programs that promise only to help children or youth get in touch with their feelings. The purpose of good treatment is, more often, to learn to control behavior and modify emotional reactions.

Parents should ask questions about the frequency at which restraints and put-downs are used and the level and type of medications that are routinely prescribed. Child abuse has occurred in treatment facilities. Children with uninvolved parents and no advocates are at risk for maltreatment. The attitude of the staff toward clients must be discerned. Children thrive in systems that are loving and nurturing, not in oppressive, punishing environments.

Roles

The single most important part of any out-of-home treatment plan may be the discharge plan. A good residential program begins planning for release immediately. This plan involves consultation with the many systems that may be involved with the young person. A coordinator should be available who assembles and monitors representatives from each system interacting with child. A case manager, case coordinator, or client advocate is a necessity. Parents must have one person who can explain the treatment plan and progress.

Community Programs

Community members, including families and businesses, can be involved in creating safe environments for children. The programs described next have not been well evaluated, but all have had promising results in communities that have attempted efforts to create networks of care for troubled youth.

Helping Hand Programs

In many communities, the problem of school violence spills out of the school building into the surrounding neighborhood. Assaults, sometimes with weapons, are now increasingly reported. When such violence occurs on the way to or from school, a climate of fear is created and can reduce attendance. Even when extra police are assigned to school areas, problems persist.

Helping Hand programs were initiated in Indianapolis, Indiana, in the middle 1960s as a citizen participation effort to increase the safety of youngsters traveling to and from school. Since then, such programs have been adopted by many schools and neighborhoods nationwide.

Private homes and businesses put placards in their windows exhibiting a large handprint. Children are taught in schools and through community education programs that they can go to places showing the "helping hand" when they are being teased, attacked, or intimidated. The adults in the home or business have committed themselves to assisting the children.

The programs have evolved to include careful security checks on Helping Hand volunteers. Schools or Helping Hand associations solicit parents or businesses who are both willing to help and to be investigated by the police.

By way of informal evaluation, it is clear that the program has expanded greatly since its inception. Many schools report that children feel less anxious about their walks to school and that incidents to and from school have decreased.

Restitution Programs

The old adage that punishment should fit the crime has been enacted in programs throughout the nation, attempting to teach young people the impact of their criminal actions. A common reaction to delinquency is to incarcerate the delinquent, whether in a prison or youth development center—a practice repeatedly shown to be ineffective in reducing delinquent behavior. A serious weakness of imprisonment has been that "Victims are not compensated, and offenders are not rehabilitated. Juveniles may be left with the impression that their crimes have no consequences, thus reinforcing antisocial behavior" (National School Resource Network, 1980, pp. 23–31).

Restitution programs have developed as an attempt to provide a more meaningful response to youth crime. In such programs, offenders may be required to make restitution (in the form of cash and/or services) to the victims of their crimes. Authorities may connect youngsters with jobs that will provide them with the funds they need to repay victims. For example, a young person may be placed in a community job such as working to improve parks with a sizable portion of his or her wages deducted for restitution payment.

Young people may also pay their debts in services. For example, in such programs (sometimes called "earn-it" programs) young vandals may be required to repair or clean the areas they damaged under the supervision of a custodian. This may entail painting, washing, fixing windows, or working on the very areas they defaced or destroyed. Such programs may be most effective with fairly young or first-time offenders.

Anecdotal reports of the results of restitution programs are promising. Many of the young people keep the jobs they've been assigned even after they have repaid their debts. Many districts have reported a decrease in property loss when young people were confronted directly with replacing stolen items.

Adopt-a-School and Ventures in Partnership Programs

As educational budgets shrink nationwide, the need for comprehensive school services continue to increase. Children have fewer and fewer adult resources (as the number of two-worker and single-parent families increases and the number of teachers with family responsibilities grows). Many schools have attempted to capture resources from businesses, service organizations, and industries by initiating programs that pair a school with one of these community systems. The essence of these programs is the involvement of a business or service organization and school in some mutually beneficial arrangement. Early conceptualizations anticipated that businesses would "give" to schools. As the programs have matured, many adopters or partners have realized they can learn from a group of educators and young people, just as the children and school personnel can learn from the community organizations.

Young people benefit through hands-on involvement with business practices, industrial equipment, or adult tutors, while the community organizations learn about cooperative teaming, objectives-based efforts, and effective training strategies. The components of the cooperative efforts have been very diverse, but reports from many districts indicate that some students show an increase in both skills and enthusiasm for learning.

These programs have not been developed with aggressive young people in mind, but clearly children can benefit from the involvement of positive adult models. In fact, the mere presence of supervising adults is likely to reduce aggressive acts. Further, positive role models may be quite influential in helping youth develop more hopeful life scripts for themselves.

A FINAL WORD

American society is violent, and schools are an unfortunate reflection of this fact. But when families are victimized by poverty, dangerous neighborhoods, and poor parenting skills, their communities can galvanize resources to counter the notion that the biggest and meanest are the best. Communities and families can be sources of energy, ideas, materials, and support that combine with schools' efforts to combat school violence.

Why, then, do some communities rise to the challenge of dealing with dangerous environments and young people while others seem powerless to influence their situations? We don't know the answer. We do know that while no one institution can be singularly responsible for societal change, schools (perhaps by default) are in a powerful position to influence families and community organizations. The agenda is clear. Their will to nurture extended and extensive relationships with families and the community is absolutely necessary.

References

Abadinsky, H. (1979). *Social service in criminal justice.* Englewood Cliffs, NJ: Prentice-Hall.

Abikoff, H. (1985). Efficacy of cognitive training in hyperactive children: A critical review. *Clinical Psychology Review, 5,* 479–512.

Adams, G. R. (1973). Classroom aggression: Determinants, controlling mechanisms, and guidelines for the implementation of a behavior modification program. *Psychology in the Schools, 10,* 155–168.

Adkins, W. R. (1970). Life skills: Structured counseling for the disadvantaged. *Personnel and Guidance Journal, 49,* 108–116.

Agras, W. S. (1967). Transfer during systematic desensitization therapy. *Behaviour Research and Therapy, 5,* 193–199.

Albee, G. W., & Joffe, J. M. (Eds.). (1977). *The issues: An overview of primary prevention.* Hanover, NH: University Press of New England.

Alexander, F. M. (1969). *The resurrection of the body.* New York: Dell.

Alexander, R. N., Kroth, R. L., Simpson, R. L., & Poppelreiter, T. (1982). The parent role in special education. In R. L. McDowell, G. W. Adamson, & F. W. Wood (Eds.), *Teaching emotionally disturbed children* (pp. 300–316). New York: Little, Brown.

Allen, G. J., Chinsky, J. M., Larsen, S. W., Lochman, J. E., & Selinger, H. V. (1976). *Community psychology and the schools: A behaviorally oriented multilevel of preventive approach.* Hillsdale, NJ: Erlbaum.

Allen, K. E., Hart, B., Buell, J. S., Harris, F. R., & Wolf, M. M. (1964). Effects of social reinforcement on isolate behavior of a nursery school child. *Child Development, 35,* 511–518.

Allen, K. E., Kenke, L. B., Harris, F. R., Baer, D. M., & Reynolds, N. J. (1967). Control of hyperactivity by social reinforcement of attending behavior. *Journal of Educational Psychology, 58, 231*–237.

Allison, T. S., & Allison, S. L. (1971). Time-out from reinforcement: Effect on sibling aggression. *Psychological Record, 21,* 81–88.

Allport, F. H. (1924). *Social psychology.* New York: Houghton Mifflin.

American Humane Society. (1986). *The national study of child neglect and abuse reporting.* Denver: Author.

American School Health Association. (1989). *National adolescent student health survey.* Oakland, CA: Third Party.

Anderson, L. M., Evertson, C. M., & Emmer, E. T. (1980). Dimensions in classroom management derived from recent research. *Journal of Curriculum Studies, 12,* 343–356.

Anderson, R. A. (1978). *Stress power.* New York: Human Sciences Press.

Apter, S. J. (1977). Applications of ecological theory: Toward a community special education model for troubled children. *Exceptional Children, 43,* 366–373.

Apter, S. J. (1982). *Troubled children: Troubled systems.* New York: Pergamon Press.

Apter, S. J., & Conoley, J. C. (1984). *Childhood behavior disorders and emotional disturbance: Teaching troubled children.* Englewood Cliffs, NJ: Prentice-Hall.

Arbuthnot, J., & Gordon, D. A. (1983). Moral reasoning development in correctional intervention. *Journal of Correctional Education, 34,* 133–138.

Argyle, M., Trower, P., & Bryant, B. K. (1974). Explorations in the treatment of personality disorders and neuroses by social skill training. *British Journal of Medical Psychology, 47,* 63–72.

Argyle, M. Furnham, A. & Graham, J. (1981). *Social situations.* Cambridge, England: Cambridge University Press.

Arkowitz, H., Lichtenstein, E., McGovern, K., & Hines, P. (1975). The behavioral assessment of social competence in males. *Behavior Therapy, 6,* 3–13.

Aronson, E., Blaney, N., Stephan, C., Sikes, J., & Snapp, M. (1978). *The jigsaw classroom.* Beverly Hills, CA: Sage.

Asarnow, J. R., & Meichenbaum, D. (1979). Verbal rehearsal and serial recall: The mediation training of kindergarten children. *Child Development, 50,* 1173–1177.

Assagioli, R. (1973). *The act of will.* New York: Viking Press.

Axelrod, S., & Apsche, J. (Eds.). (1982). *The effects and side effects of punishment on human behavior.* New York: Academic Press.

Ayllon, T., & Michael, J. (1959). The psychiatric nurse as a behavioral engineer. *Journal of the Experimental Analysis of Behavior, 2,* 323–334.

Ayllon, T., & Azrin, N. H. (1968). *The token economy: A motivational system for therapy rehabilitation.* New York: Appleton-Century-Crofts.

Ayoub, C., & Jacewitz, M. M. (1982). Families at risk of poor parenting: A descriptive study of sixty at risk families in a model prevention program. *Child Abuse and Neglect, 6,* 413–422.

Azrin, H. H., & Holz, W. C. (1966). Punishment. In W. K. Honig (Ed.), *Operant behavior: Areas of research and application.* New York: Appleton-Century-Crofts.

Bachrach, A. J., Erwin, W. J., & Mohr, J. P. (1965). The control of eating behavior in an anorexic by operant conditioning techniques. In L. P. Ullmann & L. Krasner (Eds.), *Case studies in behavior modification.* New York: Holt, Rinehart, & Winston.

Backman, C. (1979). Epilogue: A new paradigm. In G. Ginsburg (Ed.), *Emerging strategies in social psychological research.* Chichester, England: Wiley.

Baer, R. A., Blount, R. L., Detrick, R., & Stokes, T. F. (1987). Using intermittent reinforcement to program maintenance of verbal/nonverbal correspondence. *Journal of Applied Behavior Analysis, 20,* 179–184.

Baker, R. K., & Ball, S. J. (Eds.). (1969). *Violence and the media. A staff report to the National Commission on the Causes and Prevention of Violence.* Washington, DC: U.S. Government Printing Office.

Baker, S. B., Swisher, J. D., Nadenichek, P. E., & Popowicz, C. L. (1984). Measured effects of primary prevention strategies. *Personnel and Guidance Journal, 63,* 459–463.

Bales, J. (1985, October). Prevention: NIMH funds 5 approaches to excellence in prevention. *APA Monitor, 16,* 16–18.

Bandura, A. (1969). *Principles of behavior modification.* New York: Holt, Rinehart, & Winston.

Bandura, A. (1973). *Aggression: A social learning analysis.* Englewood Cliffs, NJ: Prentice-Hall.

Ban, J. R., & Ciminillo, L. M. (1977). *Violence and vandalism in public education.* Danville, IL: Interstate Printers.

Barker, R. G. (1968). *Ecological psychology: Concepts and methods for studying the environment of human behavior.* Stanford, CA: Stanford University Press.

Barker, R. G. (1978). *Habitats, environments, and human behavior.* San Francisco: Jossey-Bass.

Barker, R. G., & Gump, P. (1964). *Big school, small school: High school size and student behavior.* Stanford, CA: Stanford University Press.

Bartenieff, I., & Lewis, D. (1980). *Body movement: Coping with the environment.* New York: Gordon & Breach.

Baskin, E. J., & Hess, R. D. (1980). Does affective education work? A review of seven programs. *Journal of School Psychology, 18,* 40–50.

Bates, W. (1962). Caste, class, and vandalism. *Social Problems, 9,* 348–353.

Baumrind, D. (1975). Early socialization and adolescent competence. In S. E. Dragastin & G. H. Elder (Eds.), *Adolescence in the life cycle.* Washington, DC: Hemisphere.

Bayh, B. (1975, April). *Our nation's schools—A report card: "A" in school violence and vandalism.* Washington, DC: Preliminary report of the subcommittee to investigate juvenile delinquency, U. S. Senate.

Bayh, B. (1977). (Chairman) *Challenge for the third century—Final report on the nature and prevention of school violence and vandalism.* Washington, DC: U. S. Government Printing Office.

Bayh, B. (1978). School violence and vandalism: Problems and solutions. *Journal of Research and Development in Education, 11,* 5–9.

Beatty, F. (1977). The new model me. *American Education, 12*(1), 23–36.

Becker, W. C., Madsen, C. H., Arnold, C. R., & Thomas, D. R. (1967). The contingent use of teacher attention and praise in reducing classroom behavior problems. *Journal of Special Education, 1,* 287–307.

Beckmeyer, G. H. (1974). Rational counseling with youthful offenders. *American Journal of Correction, 6,* 34.

Berliner, D. C. (1988). Implications of studies on expertise in pedagogy for teacher education and evaluation. In *New directions for teacher assessment* (Proceedings of the 1988 ETS Invitational Conference, pp. 39–68). Princeton, NJ: Educational Testing Service.

Bernstein, P. (1975). *Theory and methods in dance–movement therapy.* Dubuque, IA: Kendall/Hunt.

Berman, P., & McLaughlin, M. W. (1976). Implementation of educational innovation. *Educational Forum, 40,* 345–370.

Berman, D. S., & Davis-Berman, J. (1991). Wilderness therapy and adolescent mental health: Administrative and clinical issues. *Administration and Policy in Mental Health, 18,* 373–379.

Bernard, M. E., & Joyce, M. R. (1984). *Rational emotive therapy with children and adolescents.* New York: Wiley.

Beverly, C. C. & Stanback, H. J. (1986). The black underclass: Theory and reality. *Black Scholar, 17,* 24–31.

Bishop, A. J., & Whitfield, R. C. (1972). *Situations in teaching.* Maidenhead, England: McGraw-Hill.

Blechman, E. A. (1985). *Solving child behavior problems at home and at school.* Champaign, IL: Research Press.

Blechman, E. A., Taylor, C. J., & Schrader, S. M. (1981). Family problem solving versus home notes as early intervention for high-risk children. *Journal of Consulting and Clinical Psychology, 49,* 919–926.

Blechman, E. A., Kotanchick, N. L., & Taylor, C. J. (1981). Families and school together: Early behavioral intervention with high risk children. *Behavior Therapy, 12,* 308–319.

Block, A. The battered teacher. (1977). *Today's Education, 66,* 58–62.

Block, A. M. (1978). Combat neurosis in inner-city schools. *American Journal of Psychiatry, 135,* 1189–1192.

Bloodworth, D. (1966). *The Chinese looking glass.* New York: Dell.

Bogardus, E. S. (1943). Gangs of Mexican-American Youth. *Sociology and Social Research, 28,* 55–66.

Boike, M. F. (1986, August). *Classroom coping skills program.* Paper presented at the annual meeting of the American Psychological Association, Washington, DC.

Bond, L. A., & Rosen, J. C. (Eds.). (1980). *Competence and coping during adulthood.* Hanover, NH: University Press of New England.

Borg, W. R., & Ascione, F. R. (1979). Changing on-task, and disruptive pupil behavior in elementary mainstreaming classrooms. *Journal of Educational Research, 72,* 243–252.

Borg, W. R., & Ascione, F. R. (1982). Classroom management in elementary mainstreaming classrooms. *Journal of Educational Psychology, 74,* 85–95.

Bostow, D. E., & Bailey, J. S. (1969). Modification of severe disruptive and aggressive behavior using brief time out and reinforcement procedures. *Journal of Applied Behavior Analysis, 2,* 31–37

Bower, E. M. (1965). Primary prevention of mental and emotional disorders. A conceptual framework and action possibilities. In N. M. Lambert (Ed.), *The protection and promotion of mental health in schools* (Public Health Service

Publication No. 1226, pp. 1–9). Bethesda, MD: U.S. Department of Health, Education, and Welfare.

Boyer, E. L. (1983). *High school: A report on secondary education in America.* New York: Harper & Row.

Bremmer, R. H. (1976). Other people's children. *Journal of Social History, 16,* 83–103.

Bresler, F. (1980). *The Chinese mafia.* New York: Stein & Day.

Brooks, C. V. W. (1974). *Sensory awareness: The rediscovery of experiencing.* New York: Viking.

Brophy, J. (1986). Teacher influences on student achievement. *American Psychologist, 41,* 1069–1077.

Brophy, J. E. (1986). Teaching and learning mathematics: Where research should be going. *Journal for Research in Mathematics Education, 17,* 323–346.

Brophy, J. E., & Putnam, J. G. (1979). Classroom management in the elementary grades. In D. L. Duke (Ed.), *Classroom management: The seventy-eighth yearbook of the National Society for the Study of Education, Part II.* Chicago: University of Chicago Press.

Brophy, J. E., & Rohrkemper, M. M. (1980a). *The influence of problem ownership on teachers' perceptions of and strategies for coping with problem students* (Research Series No. 84). East Lansing, MI: Institute for Research on Teaching, Michigan State University.

Brophy, J. E., & Rohrkemper, M. M. (1980b). *Teachers' specific strategies for dealing with hostile aggressive students* (Research Series No. 86). East Lansing, MI: Institute for Research on Teaching, Michigan State University.

Brophy, J. E., & Evertson, C. M. (1976). *Learning from teaching: A developmental perspective.* Boston: Allyn & Bacon.

Brown, P., & Elliott, R. (1965). Control of aggression in a nursery school class. *Journal of Experimental Child Psychology, 2,* 103–107.

Brown, P. & Fraser, C. (1979). Speech as a marker of situations. In K. Scherer & H. Giles (Eds.), *Social markers in speech.* Cambridge, England: Cambridge University Press.

Brown, R. (1976). *Children and television.* Newbury Park, CA: Sage.

Brown, W. K. (1978). Black gangs as family extensions. *International Journal of Offender Therapy and Comparative Criminology, 22,* 39–48.

Bryan, J. H. & Test, M. A. (1967). Models and helping: Naturalistic studies in aiding behavior. *Journal of Personality and Social Psychology, 6,* 400–407.

Bullmer, K. (1972). Improving accuracy of interpersonal perception through a direct teaching method. *Journal of Counseling Psychology, 19,* 37–41.

Bullock, L. (1983). School violence and what teachers can do about it. *Contemporary Education, 55,* 40–44.

Burchard, J. D., & Barrera, F. (1972). An analysis of time out and response cost in a programmed environment. *Journal of Applied Behavior Analysis, 5,* 271–282.

Bureau of Justice Statistics. (1992. January). *National update* (Vol. 1). Washington, DC: Author

Buss, A. H., & Plomin, R. (1984). *Temperament: Early developing personality traits.* Hillsdale, NJ: Erlbaum.

Buys, C. J. (1972). Effects of teacher reinforcement on elementary pupils' behavior and attitudes. *Psychology in the Schools, 9,* 278–288.

Calderhead, J. C. (1984). *Teachers' classroom decision making.* New York: Holt, Rinehart, & Winston.

Calhoun, K. S., & Matherne, P. (1975). The effects of varying schedules of timeout on aggressive behavior of a retarded girl. *Journal of Behavior Therapy and Experimental Psychiatry, 6,* 139–143.

California Department of Education. (1990). *School crime in California for the 1988–89 school year.* Sacramento, CA: Author.

California Youth Gang Task Force (1981). *Community access team.* Sacramento, CA: Author.

Callantine, M. F., & Warren, J. M. (1955). Learning sets in human concept formation. *Psychological Reports, 1,* 363–367.

Camp, G. M. & Camp, C. G. (1985). *Prison gangs: Their extent, nature and impact on prisons.* South Salem, NY: Criminal Justice Institute.

Canale, J. R. (1977). The effect of modeling and length of ownership on sharing behavior of children. *Social Behavior and Personality, 5,* 187–191.

Cangelosi, A., Gressard, C. F., & Mines, R. A. (1980). The effects of a rational thinking group on self-concepts of adolescents. *The School Counselor,* 357–361.

Caplan, G. (1964). *Principles of preventive psychiatry.* New York Basic Books.

Caplan, G. (1970). *The theory and practice of mental health consultation.* New York: Basic Books.

Carey, R. G., & Bucher, B. B. (1981). Identifying the educative and suppressive effects of positive practice and restitutional overcorrection. *Journal of Applied Behavior Analysis, 14,* 71–80.

Carkhuff, R. R. (1969). *Helping and human relations: A primer for lay and professional helpers: Vol. 2. Practice and research.* Amherst, MA: Human Resource Development.

Carlson, C. L., & Lahey, B. B. (1988). Conduct and attention deficit disorders. In J. C. Witt, S. N. Elliott, & F. M. Gresham (Eds.), *Handbook of behavior therapy in education.* New York: Plenum Press.

Carr, E. G. (1981). Contingency management. In A. P. Goldstein, E. G. Carr, W. Davidson, & P. Wehr, *In response to aggression.* New York: Pergamon Press.

Casey, R. J., & Berman, J. S. (1985). The outcome of psychotherapy with children. *Psychological Bulletin, 98,* 388–397.

Casserly, M. D., Bass, S. A., & Garrett, J. R. (1980). *School vandalism: Strategies for prevention.* Lexington, MA: Lexington Books.

Caught in the crossfire: A report on gun violence in our nation's schools. (1990). Washington, DC: Center to Prevent Handgun Violence.

Chandler, M. J. (1973). Egocentrism and anti-social behavior: The assessment and training of social perspective-taking skills. *Developmental Psychology, 9,* 326–332.

Chase, W. G., & Simon, H. A. (1973). Perception in chess. *Cognitive Psychology, 1,* 53–81.

Chassin, L. A., Presson, C. C., & Sherman, S. J. (1985). Stepping backward in order to step forward. *Journal of Consulting and Clinical Psychology, 52,* 612–622.

Chess, S., & Hassibi, M. (1978). *Principles and practice of child psychiatry.* New York: Plenum Press.

Christopherson, E. G., Arnold, C. M., Hill, D. W., & Quilitch, H. R. (1972). The home point system: Token reinforcement procedures for application by parents of children with behavior problems. *Journal of Applied Behavior Analysis, 5,* 485–497.

Clark, C., & Yinger, R. J. (1977). Research on teacher thinking. *Curriculum Inquiry, 7,* 280–303.

Clark, C. M., & Dunn, S. (1991). Second generation research on teachers' planning, intentions, and routines. In H. C. Waxman & H. S. Walberg (Eds.), *Effective teaching: Current research.* Berkeley, CA: McCutcheon.

Clark, C. M., & Peterson, P. L. (1986). Teachers' thought processes. In M. C. Wittrock (Ed.), *Handbook of research on teaching* (3rd ed., pp. 255–298), New York: Macmillan.

Clarke, R. V. G. (1977). Psychology and crime. *Bulletin of the British Psychological Society, 30,* 280–283.

Cleckley, H. (1964). *The mask of sanity.* St. Louis, MO: C. V. Mosby.

Cloward, R. A. & Ohlin, L. E. (1960). *Delinquency and opportunity: A theory of delinquent gangs.* New York: Free Press.

Cohen, A. K. (1955). *Delinquent boys: The culture of the gang.* New York: Free Press.

Cohen, A. K. (1966). The delinquent subculture. In R. Giallombardo (Ed.), *Juvenile delinquency.* New York: Wiley.

Cohen, J. (1969). *Statistical power analysis for the behavioral sciences.* New York: Academic Press.

Cohen, S. (1971). Direction for research on adolescent school violence and vandalism. *British Journal of Criminology, 9,* 319–340.

Colyar, D. E. (1991). Residential care and treatment of youths with conduct disorders: Conclusions of a conference of child care workers. *Child and Youth Care Forum, 20,* 195–204.

Comer, J. P. (1984). Home–school relationships as they affect the academic success of children. *Education and Urban Society, 16,* 323–337.

Comer, J. P. (1987). New Haven's school-community connection. *Educational Leadership, 44,* 13–16.

Comer, J. P. (1989). Child development and education. *Journal of Negro Education, 58,* 125–139.

Comer, J. P., & Haynes, N. M. (1991). Parent involvement in schools: An ecological approach. In Educational partnerships [Special issue]. *Elementary School Journal, 91,* 271–277.

Comstock, G. (1983). Media influences on aggression. In Center for Research Aggression (Ed.), *Prevention and control of aggression.* New York: Pergamon Press.

Cone, R. (1978). *Teachers' decisions in managing student behavior: A laboratory stimulation of interactive decision making by teachers.* Paper presented at the annual meeting of the American Educational Research Association, Toronto.

Conger, J. J., Miller, W. C., & Walsmith, C. R. (1965). Antecedents of delinquency: Personality, social class, and intelligence. In P. H. Mussen, J. J. Conger, & J. Kagen (Eds.), *Readings in child development and personality.* New York: Harper & Row.

Conoley, J. C. (1987). Families and schools: Theoretical and practical bridges. *Professional School Psychology, 2,* 191–203.

Conoley, J. C. & Conoley, C. W. (1982). *School consultation: A guide to practice and training.* New York: Pergamon Press.

Conoley, J. C., & Gutkin, T. B. (1986). School psychology: A reconceptualization of service delivery realities. In S. N. Elliott & J. Witt (Eds.), *The delivery of psychological services in schools* (pp. 393–424). Hillsdale, NJ: Erlbaum.

Conoley, J. C., & Haynes, G. (1992). Ecological perspectives. In R. D'Amato & B. Rothlisberg (Eds.), *Psychological perspectives on interventions: A case study approach to prescriptions for change.* White Plains, NY: Longman.

Corno, L. (1981). Cognitive organizing in classrooms. *Curriculum Inquiry, 11,* 359–377.

Cowen, E. (1984). Training for primary prevention in mental health. *American Journal of Community Psychology, 12,* 253–259.

Cowen, E. L. (1973). Social and community interventions. *Annual Review of Psychology, 24,* 423–472.

Cowen, E. L. (1977). Baby-steps toward primary prevention. *American Journal of Community Psychology, 5,* 1–22.

Cowen, E. L. (1980). The wooing of primary prevention. *American Journal of Community Psychology, 8,* 258–284.

Cowen, E. L. (1982). Primary prevention research: Barriers, needs and opportunities. *Journal of Prevention, 2,* 131–137.

Cowen, E. L. (1983). Primary prevention in mental health: Past, present, and future. In F. D. Felner, L. A. Jason, J. N. Moritsugu, & S. S. Farber (Eds.), *Preventive psychology: Theory, research, and practice* (pp. 11–25). New York: Pergamon Press.

Cowen, E. L., Trost, M. A., Lorion, R. P., Dorr, D., Izzo, L. D., & Isaacson, R. V. (1975). *New ways in school mental health: Early detection and prevention of school maladaption.* New York: Human Sciences Press.

Cronbach, L. J., & Snow, R. E. (1969). *Individual differences in learning ability as a function of instructional variables* (Office of Education Final Report). Stanford, CA: Stanford University Press.

Cullen, F. T., & Tinto, V. A. (1975, April). *A Mertonian analysis of school deviance.* Paper presented at the annual meeting of the American Educational Research Association, Washington, DC.

Curran, J. P. (1977). Skills training as an approach to the treatment of heterosexual-social anxiety: A review. *Psychological Bulletin, 84,* 140–157.

Davitz, D. (1964). *The communication of emotional meaning.* New York: McGraw-Hill.

DeJames, P. L. (1981). Effective parent/teacher/child relationships. *Education, 102,* 34–36.

DeLange, J. M., Lanham, S. L., & Barton, J. A. (1981). Social skills training for juvenile delinquents: Behavioral skill training and cognitive techniques. In D. Upper & S. Ross (Eds.), *Behavior group therapy* [Annual]. Champaign, IL: Research Press.

Dewey, J. (1902). *The child and the curriculum.* Chicago: University of Chicago Press.

DiGiuseppe, R. (1975). The use of behavior modification to establish rational self-statements in children. *Rational Living, 10,* 18–19.

Dil, N. (1972). *Sensitivity of emotionally disturbed and emotionally non-disturbed elementary school children to emotional meanings of facial expressions.* Unpublished doctoral dissertation, Indiana University.

Dodge, K. A., Coie, J. D., & Brakke, N. P. (1982). Behavior patterns of socially rejected and neglected preadolescents: The roles of social approach and aggression. *Journal of Abnormal Child Psychology, 10,* 389–410.

Dodge, K. A. & Murphy, R. R. (1984). The assessment of social competence in adolescents. In P. Karoly & J. J. Steffen (Eds.), *Advances in child behavior analysis and therapy* (Vol. 4). New York: Plenum Press.

Dodge, K. A., Price, J. M., Bachorowski, J., & Newman, J. P. (1990). Hostile attribution biases in severely aggressive adolescents. *Journal of Abnormal Psychology, 99,* 385–392.

Doyle, W. (1979). Making managerial decisions in classrooms. In D. L. Duke (Ed.), *Classroom managment: The seventy-eighth yearbook of the National Society for the Study of Education, Part II.* Chicago: University of Chicago Press.

Doyle, W. (1986). Classroom organization and management. In M. C. Wittrock (Ed.), *Handbook of research on teaching* (3rd ed., pp. 392–431). New York: Macmillan.

Drabman, R. S., & Spitalnik, R. (1973). Social isolation as a punishment procedure: A controlled study. *Journal of Experimental Child Psychology, 16,* 236–249.

Dreikurs, R., Grunwald, B. B., & Pepper, F. C. (1971). *Maintaining sanity in the classroom: Illustrated teaching techniques.* New York: Harper & Row.

Duke, D. L. (1976). Challenge to bureaucracy: The contemporary alternative school. *Journal of Educational Thought, 10,* 34–38.

Duke, D. L. (1978a). How administrators view the crisis in school discipline. *Phi Delta Kappan, 59,* 325–330.

Duke, D. L. (1978b). The etiology of student misbehavior and the depersonalization of blame. *Review of Educational Research, 48,* 415–437.

Duke, D. L. (1980). *Managing student behavior problems.* New York: Teachers College, Columbia University.

Duke, D. L. & Meckel, A. M. (1979). Disciplinary roles in American schools. *British Journal of Teacher Education, 6,* 37–49.

Dumpson, J. R. (1949). An approach to antisocial street gangs. *Federal Probation, 13,* 22–29.

Duncan, C. P. (1953). Transfer in motor learning as a function of degree of first-task learning and inner-task similarity. *Journal of Experimental Psychology, 45,* 1–11.

Duncan, C. P. (1958). Transfer after training with single versus multiple tasks. *Journal of Experimental Psychology, 55,* 63–72.

Durlak, J. A. (1983). Social problem-solving as a primary prevention strategy. In R. D. Felner, L. A. Jason, J. N. Moritsugu, & S. S. Farber (Eds.), *Preventive psychology: Theory, research, and practice* (pp. 31–48). New York: Pergamon Press.

Durlak, J. A. (1985). Primary prevention of school adjustment problems. *Journal of Consulting and Clinical Psychology, 53,* 623–630.

Durlak, J. A., & Jason, L. A. (1984). Preventive programs for school-aged children and adolescents. In M. C. Roberts & L. Peterson (Eds.), *Prevention of problems in childhood: Psychological research and applications* (pp. 103–132). New York: Wiley.

Eastman, B. G., & Rasbury, W. C. (1981). Cognitive self- instruction for the control of impulsive classroom behavior: Ensuring the treatment package. *Journal of Abnormal Child Psychology, 9,* 381–387.

Edgerton, S. K. (1977). Teachers in role conflict: The hidden dilemma. *Phi Delta Kappan, 59,* 120–122.

Egan, G. (1976). *Interpersonal living: A skills/contract approach to human-relations training in groups.* Pacific Grove, CA: Brooks/Cole.

Ehly, S., Conoley, J. C., Rosenthal, D. (1985). *Working with parents of exceptional students.* St. Louis, MO: Merrill.

Elardo, P. T., & Caldwell, B. M. (1979). The effects of an experimental social development program on children in the middle childhood period. *Psychology in the Schools, 16,* 93–100.

Elardo, P. T., & Cooper, M. (1977). *AWARE: Activities for social development.* Reading, MA: Addison-Wesley.

Elderly Abuse in America. (1990, May 1). *New York Times,* p. 28.

Elias, M. J., & Clabby, J. F. (1992). *Building social problem-solving skills.* San Francisco: Jossey-Bass.

Elliott, D. S., Huizinga, D., & Ageton, S. S. (1985). *Explaining delinquency and drug use.* Beverly Hills, CA: Sage.

Elliott, D. S. & Voss, H. L. (1974). *Delinquency and dropout.* Toronto: Lexington.

Elliott, S. N., Gresham, F., & Kramer, J. J. (1987). *Assessing children's problems.* New York: Little, Brown.

Ellis, A. (1973). *Humanistic psychotherapy: The rational-emotive approach.* New York: Julian Press.

Ellis, A., & Harper, R. A. (1975). *A new guide to rational living.* Englewood Cliffs, NJ: Prentice-Hall.

Ellis, H. (1965). *The transfer of learning.* New York: Macmillan.

Ellis, R. A., & Lane, W. C. (1978). Structural supports for upward mobility. *American Sociological Review, 53,* 743–756.

Ellison, W. S. (1973). School vandalism: 100 million dollar challenge. *Community Education Journal, 3,* 27–33.

Emery, J. E. (1975). *Social perception processes in normal and learning disabled children.* Unpublished doctoral dissertation, New York University.

Erikson, E. H. (1950). *Childhood and society.* New York: W. W. Norton.

Evers, W. L., & Schwartz, J. C. (1973). Modifying social withdrawal in preschoolers: The effects of filmed modeling and teacher praise. *Journal of Abnormal Child Psychology, 1,* 248–256.

Evertson, C. M., & Emmer, E. T. (1982). Effective management at the beginning of the school year in junior high classes. *Journal of Educational Psychology, 74,* 485–498.

Falk, N., & Coletti, R. F. (1982). Better vandalism protection at less cost. *American School and University, 54,* 52–54.

Farrington, D. P. (1983). Offending from 10–25 years of age. In K. T. Van Dusen & S. A. Mednick (Eds.), *Prospective studies of crime and delinquency* (pp. 17–37). Boston: Kluwer-Nijhoff.

Farrington, D. P. (1987). Early precursors of frequent offending. In J. Q. Wilson & G. C. Loury (Eds.), *From children to citizens: Vol. 3. Families, schools, and delinquency prevention* (pp. 27–51). New York: Springer-Verlag.

Farrington, D. P., Gallagher, B., Morley, L., St. Ledger, R. J., & West, D. J. (1986). *Cambridge study in delinquent development: Long term follow-up*. Unpublished annual report, Cambridge University Institute of Criminology, Cambridge, England.

Farris, R., & Dunham, H. (1939). *Mental disorders in urban areas*. Chicago: University of Chicago.

Federal Bureau of Investigation. (1989). *Uniform crime report, 1989*, Washington, DC: U.S. Government Printing Office.

Federal Bureau of Investigation. (1990). *Uniform crime report, 1990*. Washington, DC: U.S. Government Printing Office.

Federation of Child Abuse and Neglect. (1990). *Fact sheet*. New York: National Committee for Prevention of Child Abuse.

Feindler, E. L., Marriott, S. A., & Iwata, M. (1984). Group anger control training for junior high school delinquents. *Cognitive Therapy and Research, 8*, 299–311.

Feldenkrais, M. (1970). *Body and mature behavior*. New York: International Universities Press.

Feldenkrais, M. (1972). *Awareness through movement*. New York: Harper & Row.

Feldhusen, J. F. (1979). Problems of student behavior in secondary schools. In D. L. Duke (Ed.), *Classroom management* (78th yearbook of the National Society for the Study of Education, Part II). Chicago: National Society for the Study of Education.

Feldhusen, J. F., Aversano, F. M., & Thurston, J. R. (1976). Prediction of youth contacts with law enforcement agencies. *Criminal Justice and Behavior, 3*, 235–253.

Feldhusen, J. F., Roeser, T. D., & Thurston, J. R. (1977). Prediction of social adjustment over a period of six or nine years. *Journal of Special Education, 11*, 29–36.

Feldhusen, J. F., Thurston, J. R., & Benning, J. J. (1973). A longitudinal study of delinquency and other aspects of children's behavior. *International Journal of Criminology and Penology, 1, 341*–351.

Felner, R. D., Ginter, M., & Primavera, J. (1982). Primary prevention during school transitions: Social support and environmental structure. *American Journal of Community Psychology, 10*, 277–290.

Fenichel, C. (1966). Psycho-educational approaches for seriously disturbed children in the classroom. In P. Knoblock (Ed.), *Intervention approaches in educating emotionally disturbed children*. Syracuse, NY: Division of Special Education and Rehabilitation, Syracuse University.

Fenstermacher, G. D. (1979). A philosophical consideration of recent research on teacher effectiveness. In L. S. Shulman (Ed.), *Review of research in education No. 6*. Itasca, IL: Peacock.

Ferster, C. B., & DeMeyer, M. K. (1962). A method for the experimental analysis of the behavior of autistic children. *American Journal of Orthopsychiatry, 32*, 89–98.

Ferster, C. B., & Skinner, B. F. (1957). *Schedules of reinforcement.* New York: Appleton-Century-Crofts.

Feshbach, N. D. (1982). Empathy, empathy training and the regulation of aggression in elementary school children. In R. M. Kaplan, V. J. Konecni, & R. Novaco (Eds.), *Aggression in children and youth.* Alphen den Rijn, The Netherlands: Siuthogg/Noordhoff.

Feshbach, N. D., & Feshbach, S. (1969). The relationship between empathy and aggression in two age groups. *Developmental Psychology, 1,* 102–107.

Feshbach, S., & Singer, R. D. (1971). *Television and aggression: An experimental field study.* San Francisco: Jossey-Bass.

Field, T. (1981). Early peer relations. In P. S. Strain (Ed.), *The utilization of classroom peers as behavior change agents.* New York: Plenum Press.

Finkelhor, D. (1979). *Sexually victimized children.* New York: Free Press.

Firestone, P. (1976). The effects and side effects of time out on an aggressive nursery school child. *Journal of Behavior Therapy and Experimental Psychiatry, 6,* 79–81.

Fluegelman, A. (1981). *More new games.* Garden City, NY: Dolphin Books.

Fogatch, M. S., Patterson, G. R., & Skinner, M. (1990). A mediational model for the effect of divorce on antisocial behavior in boys. In E. M. Hetherington (Eds.), *The impact of divorce and step-parenting on children.* Hillsdale, NJ: Erlbaum.

Forehand, R., Roberts, M. W., Dolays, D. M., Hobbs, S. A., & Resick, P. A. (1976). An examination of disciplinary procedures with children. *Journal of Experimental Child Psychology, 21,* 109–120.

Forgays, D. G. (Ed.). (1978). *Environmental influences and strategies in primary prevention.* Hanover, NH: University Press of New England.

Foster, H. J. (1974). *Ribbin', jivin', and playin' the dozens.* Cambridge, MA: Ballinger.

Foxx, R. M., & Azrin, N. H. (1973). Restitution: A method of eliminating aggressive-disruptive behavior for retarded and brain damaged patients. *Behaviour Research and Therapy, 10,* 15–27.

Frank, S. J. (1977). *The facilitation of empathy through training in imagination.* Unpublished doctoral dissertation, Yale University, New Haven, CT.

Frease, D. E. (1973). Schools and delinquency: Some intervening processes. *Pacific Sociological Review, 16,* 426–448.

Freedman, B. J., Rosenthal, L., Donahoe, C. P., Schlundt, D. G., & McFall, R. M. (1978). A social-behavioral analysis of skill deficits in delinquent and nondelinquent adolescent boys. *Journal of Consulting and Clinical Psychology, 46,* 1448–1462.

Friedman, C. J., Mann, F., & Friedman, A. S. (1975). A profile of juvenile street gang members. *Adolescence, 40,* 563–607.

Fullan, M., & Pomfret, A. (1977). Research on curriculum and instruction implementation. *Review of Educational Research, 47,* 335–397.

Fuller, F. F., & Bown, O. H. (1975). Becoming a teacher. In K. Ryan (Ed.), *Teacher education* (74th yearbook of the National Society for the Study of Education, Part II). Chicago: University of Chicago Press.

Furnham, A., & Argyle, M. (1981). *More new games.* Garden City, NY: Dolphin Books.

Furnham, A., & Argyle, M. (1981). *The psychology of social situations.* New York: Pergamon Press.

Galassi, M. D., & Galassi, J. P. (1977). *Assert yourself!* New York: Human Sciences Press.

Galassi, J. P., & Galassi, M. D. (1984). Promoting transfer and maintenance of counseling outcomes. In S. D. Brown & R. W. Lent (Eds.), *Handbook of counseling psychology.* New York: Wiley.

Gambrill, E. D. (1977). *Behavior modification.* San Francisco: Jossey-Bass.

Gardner, S. (1983). *Street gangs.* New York: Franklin Watts.

Gaustad, M. (1990). *Gangs* (ERIC Digest No. EA52). Eugene, OR: ERIC Clearinghouse on Educational Management.

Gendlin, E. (1981). *Focusing.* New York: Bantam.

Gendlin, E. (1984). The politics of giving therapy away: Listening and focusing. In D. Larson (Ed.), *Teaching psychological skills.* Monterey, CA: Brooks/Cole.

Gesten, E. L., Rains, M. H., Rapkin, B. D., Weissberg, R. P., Flores De Apodaca, R., Cowen, E. G., & Bowen, R. (1982). Training children in social problem-solving competencies: A first and second look. *American Journal of Community Psychology, 10,* 95–115.

Giebink, J. W., Stover, D. S., & Fahl, M. A. (1968). Teaching adaptive responses to frustration to emotionally disturbed boys. *Journal of Consulting and Clinical Psychology, 32,* 336–368.

Gil, D. G. (1970). *Violence against children: Physical child abuse in the United States.* Cambridge, MA: Harvard University Press.

Gilliam, J. E., Stough, L., & Fad, K. (1991). Interventions for swearing. In G. Stoner, M. R. Shinn, & H. M. Walker (Eds.), *Interventions for achievement and behavior problems.* Silver Springs, MD: National Association of School Psychologists.

Glaser, D. (1956). Criminality theories and behavioral images. In D. R. Cressey & D. A. Ward (Eds.), *Delinquency, crime, and social process.* New York: Harper & Row.

Glaser, R. (1972). Individuals and learning: The new aptitudes. *Educational Researcher, 1,* 5–12.

Glaser, R. (1981). The future of testing: A research agenda for cognitive psychology and psychometrics. *American Psychologist, 36,* 923–936.

Glasgow, D. G. (1980). *The black underclass: Poverty, unemployment, and entrapment of ghetto youth.* San Francisco: Jossey-Bass.

Glass, G. V., Cahen, L. S., Smith, M. L., & Filby, N. N. (1982). *School class size: Research and policy.* Beverly Hills, CA: Sage.

Glasser, W. (1969). *Schools without failure.* New York: Harper & Row.

Glick, B., & Goldstein, A. P. (1987). Aggression replacement training. *Journal of Counseling and Development, 65,* 356–362.

Glidewell, J. C., Gildea, M. C., & Kaufman, M. K. (1973). The preventive and therapeutic effects of two school mental health programs. *American Journal of Community Mental Health, 1,* 295–329.

Glueck, S., & Glueck, E. (1940). *Juvenile delinquents grown up.* New York: Commonwealth Fund.

Gnagey, W. J. (1968). *The psychology of discipline in the classroom.* New York: Macmillan.

Gold, M. (1978). Scholastic experiences, self-esteem, and delinquent behavior: A theory for alternative schools. *Crime and Delinquency,* 290–309.

Goldman, N. (1961). A socio-psychological study of school vandalism. *Crime and Delinquency, 7,* 221–230.

Goldmeir, H. (1974). Vandalism: The effects and unmanageable confrontatons. *Adolescence, 9,* 49–56.

Goldstein, A. P. (Ed.). (1978). *Prescriptions for child mental health and education.* New York: Pergamon Press.

Goldstein, A. P. (1981). *Psychological skill training.* New York: Pergamon Press.

Goldstein, A. P. (1988). *The prepare curriculum.* Champaign, IL: Research Press.

Goldstein, A. P. (1991). *Delinquent gangs: A psychological perspective.* Champaign, IL: Research Press.

Goldstein, A. P., Apter, S. J., & Harootunian, B. (1984). *School violence.* Englewood Cliffs, NJ: Prentice-Hall.

Goldstein, A. P., & Glick, B. (1987). *Aggression replacement training: A comprehensive intervention for aggressive youth.* Champaign, IL: Research Press.

Goldstein, A. P., Glick, B., Irwin, M. J., Pask, C., & Rubama. I. (1989). *Reducing delinquency: Intervention in the community.* New York: Pergamon Press.

Goldstein, A. P., & Kanfer, F. (1979). *Maximizing treatment gains: Transfer enhancement in psychotherapy.* New York: Academic Press.

Goldstein, A. P., Keller, H., & Erne, D. (1985). *Changing the abusive parent.* Champaign, IL: Research Press.

Goldstein, A. P., Lopez, M., & Greenleaf, D. M. (1979). Introduction. In A. P. Goldstein & F. H. Kanfer (Eds.), *Maximizing treatment gains.* New York: Academic Press.

Goldstein, A. P., & Michaels, G. Y. (1985). *Empathy: Development, training and consequences.* Hillsdale, NJ: Erlbaum.

Goldstein, A. P., Monti, P. J., Sardino, T. J., & Green, D. J. (1979). *Police crisis intervention.* New York: Pergamon Press.

Goldstein, A. P., & Pentz, M. A. (1984). Psychological skill training and the aggressive adolescent. *School Psychology Review, 13,* 311–323.

Goldstein, A. P., & Rosenbaum. A. (1982). *Aggress-less.* Englewood Cliffs, NJ: Prentice-Hall.

Goldstein, A. P., & Segall, M. (1983). *Aggression in global perspective.* New York: Pergamon Press.

Goldstein, A. P., Sherman, M., Gershaw, N. J., Sprafkin, R. P., & Glick, B. (1978). Training aggressive adolescents in prosocial behavior. *Journal of Youth and Adolescence, 7,* 73–92.

Goldstein, A. P., Sprafkin, R. P., Gershaw, N. J., & Klein, P. (1980). *Skillstreaming the adolescent.* Champaign, IL: Research Press.

Goldstein, A. P., & Stein, N. (1976). *Prescriptive psychotherapies.* New York: Pergamon Press.

Goldston, S. E. (1986). Primary prevention: Historical perspectives and a blueprint for action. *American Psychologist, 41,* 453–460.

Goleman, D. (1977). *The varieties of the meditative experience.* New York: Dutton.

Good, T. L., & Brophy, J. E. (1978). *Looking in classrooms.* New York: Harper & Row.

Good, T. L., & Weinstein, R. S. (1986). Schools make a difference: Evidence, criticisms, and new directions. *American Psychologist, 41,* 1090–1097.

Goodlad, J. I. (1984). *A place called school: Prospects for the future.* New York: McGraw-Hill.

Gordon, E. W. (1982). Human ecology and the mental health professions. *American Journal of Orthopsychiatry, 52,* 109–110.

Gordon, E. W. (1982). Human ecology and the mental health profesisons. *American Journal of Orthopsychiatry, 52,* 109–110.

Gott, R. (1989, May). *Juvenile gangs.* Paper presented at the Conference on Juvenile Crime, Eastern Kentucky University.

Gough, H. G. (1948). A sociological theory of psychopathy. *American Journal of Sociology, 53,* 359–366.

Grant, C. A. (1989). Equity, equality and classroom life. In W. G. Secada (Ed.), *Equity in education* (pp. 89–102). London: Falmer Press.

Grant, C. A., & Secada, W. C. (1990). Preparing teachers for diversity. In W. R. Houston (Ed.), *Handbook of research on teacher education* (pp. 403–422). New York: Macmillan.

Grant, J. E. (1987). *Problem solving intervention for aggressive adolescent males: A preliminary investigation.* Unpublished doctoral dissertation, Syracuse University, Syracuse, NY.

Gray, E. B. (1983). *Final Report: Collaborative research of community and minority group action to prevent child abuse and neglect: Vol. I. Perinatal interventions.* Chicago: National Committee for Prevention of Child Abuse.

Gray, J., Cutler, C., Dean, J., & Kempe, C. H. (1976). Perinatal assessment of mother–baby interaction. In R. E. Helfer & C. H. Kempe (Eds.), *Child abuse and neglect: The family and the community* (pp. 377–392). Chicago: University of Chicago Press.

Gray, K. C., & Hutchison, H. C. (1964). The psychopathic personality: A survey of Canadian psychiatrists' opinions. *Canadian Psychiatric Association Journal, 9,* 452–461.

Gray, J., & Kaplan, B. (1980). The lay health visitor program: An eighteen month experience. In C. H. Kempe & R. Helfer (Eds.), *The battered child* (pp. 363–378). Chicago: University of Chicago Press.

Gray, S. W., & Wandersman, L. P. (1980). The methodology of home-based intervention studies: Problems and promising strategies. *Child Development, 51,* 993–1009.

Greenberg, B. (1969). *School vandalism: A national dilemma.* Menlo Park, CA: Stanford Research Institute.

Greenberg, B. (1974). School vandalism: Its effects and paradoxical solutions. *Crime Prevention Review, 1,* 11–18.

Greenwood, C. R., Hops, H., Delquadri, J., & Guild, J. (1974). Group contingencies for group consequences in classroom management: A further analysis. *Journal of Applied Behavior Analysis, 7,* 413–425.

Gruber, R. P. (1971). Behavior therapy: Problems in generalization. *Behavior Therapy, 2*, 361–368.

Guerney, B. G. (1977). *Relationship enhancement: Skill training programs for therapy, problem-prevention, and enrichment.* San Francisco: Jossey-Bass.

Gump, P. V. (1980). The school as a social situation. *Annual Review of Psychology, 31*, 553–582.

Gump, P. V. (1982). School settings and their keeping. In D. L. Duke (Ed.), Helping teachers manage classrooms (pp. 98–114). Alexandria, VA: Association for Supervision and Curriculum Development.

Gunther, B. (1968). *Sense relaxation below your mind.* New York: Collier.

Guralnick, M. J. (1981). Peer influences on the development of communicative competence. In P. Strain (Ed.), *The utilization of classroom peers as behavior change agents.* New York: Plenum Press.

Guttman, E. S. (1970). Effects of short-term psychiatric treatment for boys in two California Youth Authority institutions. In D. C. Gibbons (Ed.), *Delinquent behavior.* Englewood Cliffs, NJ: Prentice-Hall.

Hagebak, R. (1979). Disciplinary practices in Dallas. In D. G. Gil (Ed.), *Child abuse and violence.* New York: AMS Press.

Hagedorn, J. & Macon, P. (1988). *People and folks.* Chicago: Lake View Press.

Hall, R. V., Axelrod, S., Foundopoulos, M., Shellman, J., Campbell, R. A., & Cranston, S. S. (1971). The effective use of punishment to modify behavior in the classroom. *Educational Technology, 11*, 24–26.

Hall, R. V., Lund, D., & Jackson, D. (1968). Effects of teacher attention on study behavior. *Journal of Applied Behavior Analysis, 1*, 1–12.

Hall, R. V., Panyan, M., Rabon, D., & Broden, M. (1968). Instructing beginning teachers in reinforcement procedures which improve classroom control. *Journal of Applied Behavior Analysis, 1*, 315–322.

Hansford, B. C., & Hattie, J. A. (1982). The relationship between self and achievement/performance measures. *Review of Educational Research, 52*, 123–142.

Hardman, D. G. (1967). Historical perspectives on gang research. *Journal of Research in Crime and Delinquency, 4*, 5–27.

Hare, M. A. (1976, March). *Teaching conflict resolution situations.* Paper presented at the meeting of the Eastern Community Association, Philadelphia.

Harootunian, B. (1980). Teacher effectiveness: The view from within. *Theory into Practice, 19*, 266–270.

Harootunian, B. (1986). School violence and vandalism. In A. P. Goldstein & S. J. Apter (Eds.), *Youth violence: Programs and prospects* (pp. 120–139). New York: Pergamon Press.

Harootunian, B., & Apter, S. J. (1983). Violence in school. In A. P. Goldstein (Ed.), *Prevention and control of aggression* (pp. 66–83). New York: Pergamon Press.

Harootunian, B., & Yarger, G. (1981). *Teachers' conceptions of their own success.* Washington, DC: ERIC Clearinghouse on Teacher Education.

Harre, R., & Secord, P. F. (1972). *The explanation of social behaviour.* Oxford, England: Basil Blackwell.

Harris, J. D., Gray, B. A., Rees-McGee, S. R., Carroll, J. L., & Zaremba, E. T. (1987). Referrals to school psychologists: A national survey. *Journal of School Psychology, 25*, 343–354.

Harris, J. W. (1981). Cramping your arsonist's style and cutting energy costs — All by computer. *Thrust for Educational Leadership, 11,* 18–19.

Harris, V. W., & Sherman, J. A. (1973). Effects of peer tutoring and consequences on the math performance of elementary school classroom students. *Journal of Applied Behavior Analysis, 6,* 587–597.

Hauck, P. (1967). *The rational management of children.* New York: Libra.

Hawkins, J. D., & Fraser, M. W. (1983). Social support networks in delinquency prevention and treatment. In J. K. Wittaker & J. Garbarino (Eds.), *Social support networks.* New York: Aldine.

Hawley, R. C., & Hawley, I. L. (1975). *Developing human potential: A handbook of activities for personal and social growth.* Amherst, MA: Educational Research Associates.

Heffernan, J. A., & Albee, G. W. (1985). Prevention perspectives from Vermont to Washington. *American Psychologist, 40,* 202–204.

Heil, L. M., Powell, M., & Feifer, I. (1960). *Characteristics of teachers' behavior related to the achievement of children in several elementary grades* (Cooperative Research Project No. 352, Mimeographed). Brooklyn, NY: Brooklyn College.

Heiman, H. (1973). Teaching interpersonal communications. *North Dakota Speech and Theatre Association Bulletin, 2,* 7–29.

Helfer, R. E., & Kempe, C. H. (Eds.). (1976). *The battered child.* Chicago: University of Chicago Press.

Hellman, D. A., & Beaton, S. (1986). The pattern of violence in urban public schools: The influence of school and community. *Journal of Research in Crime and Delinquency, 23,* 102–127.

Helmreich, W. B. (1973). Race, sex and gangs. *Society, 11,* 44–50.

Henker, B., & Whalen, C. K. (1989). Hyperactivity and attention deficits. *American Psychologist, 44,* 216–223.

Hightower, A. D., & Avery, R. R. (1986, August). *The study buddy program.* Paper presented at the annual meeting of the American Psychological Association, Washington, DC.

Hirschi, T. (1969). *Causes of delinquency.* Berkeley: University of California Press.

Hobbs, N. (1966). Helping disturbed children: Psychological and ecological strategies. *American Psychologist, 21,* 1105–1115.

Hobbs, N. (1975). *The futures of children.* San Francisco: Jossey-Bass.

Hofer, M. (1978). *Implicit personality theory of teachers, causal attribution, and their perception of students.* Paper presented at the annual meeting of the American Educational Research Association, Toronto.

Homme, L. (1971). *How to use contingency contracting in the classroom.* Champaign, IL: Research Press.

Horowitz, R. (1983). *Honor and the American dream.* New Brunswick, NJ: Rutgers University Press.

Howard, A., & Scott, R. A. (1981). The study of minority groups in complex societies. In R. H. Monroe, R. L. Monroe, & B. B. Whiting (Eds.), *Handbook of cross-cultural human development.* New York: Garland STPM Press.

Howard, J. L. (1978). Factors in school vandalism. *Journal of Research and Development in Education, 11,* 13–18.

Howitt, D., & Cumberbatch, G. (1975). *Violence and the mass media.* London: Paul Elek.

Hughes, J. N., & Baker, D. B. (1990). *The clinical child interview.* New York: Guilford Press.

Hunt, D. E. (1971). *Matching models in education.* Toronto: Ontario Institute for Studies in Education.

Hunt, D. E. (1975). Person-environment interaction: A challenge found wanting before it was tried. *Review of Educational Research, 45,* 209-230(a).

Hunt, D. E. (1976). Teachers' adaptation: 'Reading' and 'flexing' to students. *Journal of Teacher Education, 27,* 268-275.

Hunt, D. E. (1977). Theory to practice as persons-in-relation. *Ontario Psychologist, 9,* 52-62.

Hunt, D. E. (1980). How to be your own best theorist. *Theory into Practice, 19,* 287-293.

Hunt, D. E. (1987). *Beginning with ourselves.* Cambridge: MA: Brookline.

Hunt, D. E., & Sullivan, E. V. (1974). *Between psychology and education.* Hinsdale, IL: Dryden Press.

Hutton, J. B. (1985). What reasons are given by teachers who refer problem behavior students. *Psychology in the schools, 22,* 79-82.

Hyman, I. A. (1978). Is the hickory stick out of tune? *Today's Education, 2,* 30-32.

Ianni, F. A. J. (1978). The social organization of the high school: School-specific aspects of school crime. In E. Wenk & N. Harlow (Eds.), *School crime and disruption.* Davis, CA: Responsible Action.

Idol, L., & West, J. F. (1987). Consultation in special education (Part 2): Training and practice. *Journal of Learning Disabilities, 20,* 474-494.

Inciardi, J. A., & Pottieger, A. E. (1978). (Eds). *Violent crime: Historical and contemporary issues.* Beverly Hills, CA: Sage.

Ivey, A. E., & Authier, J. (1971). *Microcounseling.* Springfield, IL: C. C. Thomas.

Iwata, B. A. (1987). Negative reinforcement in applied behavior analysis: An emerging technology. *Journal of Applied Behavior Analysis, 20,* 361-378.

Jackson, D. A., Della-Piana, G. M., & Sloane, H. N. (1975). *How to establish a behavior observation system.* Englewood Cliffs, NJ: Educational Technology.

Jackson, P. (1968). *Life in classrooms.* New York: Holt, Rinehart. & Winston.

Jacobson, E. (1964). *Anxiety and tension control.* Philadelphia: J. B. Lippincott.

Jason, L. A., Durlak, J. A., & Holton-Walker, E. (1984). Prevention of child problems in the schools. In M. C. Roberts & L. Peterson (Eds.), *Prevention of problems in childhood: Psychological research and applications* (pp. 311-341). New York: Wiley.

Jason, L. A., Frasure, S., & Ferone, L. (1981). Establishing supervising behaviors in eighth graders and peer-tutoring behaviors in first graders. *Child Study Journal, 11,* 201-219.

Jessor, R. J., & Jessor, S. L. (1977). *Problem behavior and psychosocial development.* New York: Academic Press.

Johnson, D. W., & Johnson, R. T. (1975). *Learning together and alone.* Englewood Cliffs, NJ: Prentice-Hall.

Johnson, D. W., & Johnson, R. T. (1988). *Cooperation in the classroom.* Edina, MN: Interaction Book.

Jones, F. H., & Miller, W. H. (1974). The effective use of negative attention for reducing group disruption in special elementary school classrooms. *Psychological Record, 24,* 435–448.

Jones, R. R., Weinrott, M. R., & Howard, J. R. (1981). *The national evaluation of the Teaching Family Model.* Eugene, OR: Evaluation Research Group.

Jones, M. (1953). *The therapeutic community.* New York: Basic Books.

Joyce, B. (1978–1979). Toward a theory of information processing in teaching. *Educational Research Quarterly, 3,* 66–67.

Joyce, B. R., & Harootunian, B. (1967). *The structure of teaching.* Chicago: Science Research Associates.

Judd, C. H. (1902). The relation of special training to general intelligence. *Educational Review, 36,* 28–42.

Juul, K. D. (1977, July). *Educational and psychological interactions: Models of remediation for behavior disordered children* (Bulletin No. 62). Malmo, Sweden: Department of Education and Psychological Research, School of Education.

Kagan, S. (1985). Learning to cooperate. In R. Slavin, S. Sharan, S. Kagan, R. Hertz-Lazarowtiz, C. Webb, & R. Schmuck (Eds.), *Learning to cooperate, cooperating to learn.* New York: Plenum.

Kanfer, F. H., & Goldstein, A. P. (1991). *Helping people change* (4th ed.). New York: Pergamon Press.

Kaplan, D. E., & Dubro, A. (1986). *Yakuza: The explosive account of Japan's criminal underworld.* Reading, MA: Addison-Wesley.

Karoly, P. (1980). Operant methods. In F. Kanfer & A. P. Goldstein (Eds.), *Helping people change.* New York: Pergamon Press.

Karoly, P., & Steffen, J. J. (Eds.). (1980). *Improving the long-term effects of psychotherapy.* New York: Gardner.

Kauffman, C., Grunebaum, H., Cohler, B. J., & Gamer, E. (1979). Superkids: Competent children of psychotic mothers. *American Journal of Psychiatry, 136,* 1398–1402.

Kaufman, K. F., & O'Leary, K. D. (1972). Reward, cost, and self-evaluation procedures for disruptive adolescents in a psychiatric hospital school. *Journal of Applied Behavior Analysis, 5,* 293–310.

Kazdin, A. E. (1975). *Behavior modification in applied settings.* Homewood, IL: Dorsey Press.

Kazdin, A. E. (1977). *The token economy.* New York: Plenum Press.

Kazdin, A. E. (1987). *Conduct disorders in childhood and adolescence* (Vol. 9). Beverly Hills, CA: Sage.

Kazdin, A. E. (1987). Treatment of antisocial behavior in children: Current status and future direction. *Psychological Bulletin, 102,* 187–203.

Kazdin, A. E. (1989). *Behavior modification in applied settings* (4th ed.). Pacific Grove, CA: Brooks/Cole.

Kazdin, A. E. (1989). Developmental psychopathology: Current research, issues, and directions. *American Psychologist, 44,* 180–187.

Keeley, S. M., Shemberg, K. M., & Carbonell, J. (1976). Operant clinical intervention: Behavior management or beyond? Where are the data? *Behavior Therapy, 7,* 292–305.

Keiser, R. L. (1969). *The Vice Lords: Warriors of the streets.* New York: Holt, Rinehart, & Winston.

Kelly, D. H. (1975). Status origins, track positions, and delinquent involvement. *Sociological Quarterly, 12,* 65–85.

Kelly, G. A. (1955). *The psychology of personal constructs* (Vol. 1). New York: W. W. Norton.

Keen, S. (1970, October). Sing the body electric. *Psychology Today,* pp. 56–61.

Kempe, C. H., Silverman, F. N., Steele, B. F., Droegemueller, W., & Silver, H. K. (1962). The battered child syndrome. *Journal of the American Medical Association, 181,* 17–24.

Kendall, P. C. (1985). Toward a cognitive–behavioral model of child psychopathology and a critique of related interventions. *Journal of Abnormal Child Psychology, 13,* 357–372.

Kent, M. W., & Rolf, J. E. (1979). (Eds.). *Social competence in children.* Hanover, NH: University Press of New England.

Kerr, M., Strain, P., & Ragland, E. (1982). Teacher-mediated peer feedback treatment of behaviorally handicapped children. *Behavior Modification, 6,* 277–290.

Kirschenbaum, D. S., & Ordman, A. M. (1984). Preventive interventions for children: Cognitive behavioral perspectives. In A. W. Meyers & W. E. Craighead (Eds.), *Cognitive–behavioral therapy with children* (pp. 377–409). New York: Plenum Press.

Kirschner, N. M., & Levin, L. (1975). A direct school intervention program for the modification of aggressive behavior. *Psychology in the Schools, 12,* 202–208.

Klaus, M. H., & Kennell, J. H. (1976). *Maternal–infant bonding.* St. Louis, MO: C. V. Mosby.

Klein, M. W. (1971). *Street gangs and street workers.* Englewood Cliffs, NJ: Prentice-Hall.

Klein, M. W. (1968). *The Ladino Hills Project* (Final report to the Office of Juvenile Delinquency and Youth Development). Washington, DC: Office of Juvenile Delinquency and Youth Development.

Klein, M. W., Maxson, C. L. (1989). Street gang violence. In N. A. Weiner & N. W. Wolfgang (Eds.), *Violent crime, violent criminals.* Newbury Park, CA: Sage.

Kluckhohn, C., & Murray, H. A. (Eds.). (1949). *Personality in nature, society, and culture.* New York: Knopf.

Knaus, W. (1974). *Rational–emotive education: A manual for elementary school teachers.* New York: Institute for Rational Living.

Knaus, W., & Boker, S. (1975). The effect of rational-emotive education lessons on anxiety and self-concept in sixth-grade children. *Rational Living, 11,* 7–10.

Knight, B. J., & West, D. J. (1975). Temporary and continuing delinquency. *British Journal of Criminology, 15,* 43–50.

Kobrin, S. (1959). The Chicago Area Project: A twenty-five year assessment. *Annals of the American Academy of Political and Social Science, 322,* 136–151.

Kochman, T. (1981). *Black and White styles in conflict.* Chicago: University of Chicago Press.

Kodluboy, D. W., & Evenrud, L. A. (1993). School-based interventions: Best practices and critical issues. In A. P. Goldstein & C. R. Huff (Eds.), *The gang intervention handbook.* Champaign, IL: Research Press.

Kohlberg, L. (1969). Stage and sequence: The cognitive- developmental approach to socialization. In D. A. Goslin (Ed.), *Handbook of socialization theory and research.* Chicago: Rand McNally.

Kohlberg, L. (Ed.). (1973). *Collected papers on moral development and moral education.* Cambridge, MA: Center for Moral Education, Harvard University.

Kounin, J. S. (1970). *Discipline and group management in classrooms.* New York: Holt, Rinehart, & Winston.

Kounin, J. S. (1975). An ecological approach to classroom activity settings: Some methods and findings. In R. Weinberg and R. Wood (Eds.), *Observation of pupils and teachers in mainstream and special education settings: Alternative strategies.* Minneapolis: Leadership Training Institute.

Ladd, G. W., & Mize, J. (1983). A cognitive–social learning model of social skill training. *Psychological Review, 90,* 127–157.

Landesco, J. (1932). Crime and the failure of institutions in Chicago's immigrant areas. *Journal of Criminal Law and Criminology,* July, 238–248.

Larkin, J., McDermott, J., Simon, D. P., & Simon, H. A. (1980). Expert and novice performance in solving physics problems. *Science, 208,* 1335–1342.

Lazar, I., & Darlington, R. (1982). Lasting effects of early education: A report from the consortium for longitudinal studies. *Monograph of the Society for Research in Child Development, 47*(2–3), Serial No. 195.

Lazarus, A. A., & Rachman, S. (1967). The use of systematic desensitization in psychotherapy. *South African Medical Journal, 31,* 934–937.

Lefkowitz, M. M., Eron, L., Walder, L. O., & Huessman, L. R. (1977). Television violence and child aggression. In G. A. Comstock, E. A. Rubenstein, & J. P. Murray (Eds.), *Television and social behavior* (Vol. 3). Washington, DC: U.S. Government Printing Office.

Leftwich, D. (1977). *A study of vandalism in selected public schools in Alabama.* Unpublished doctoral dissertation, University of Alabama, Tuscaloosa.

Leitenberg, H., Agras, W. S., & Thomson, L. E. (1968). A sequential analysis of the effect of selective positive reinforcement in modifying anorexia nervosa. *Behaviour Research and Therapy, 6,* 211–218.

Lentz, F. E. (1988). Reductive procedures. In J. C. Witt, S. N. Elliott, & F. M. Gresham (Eds.), *Handbook of behavior therapy in education.* New York: Plenum Press.

Lentz, F. E., & Shapiro, E. S. (1986). Functional assessment of the academic environment. *School Psychology Review, 15,* 346–357.

Lesh, T. V. (1970). Zen meditation and the development of empathy in counselors. *Journal of Humanistic Psychology, 10,* 39–74.

Lewin, K. (1951). *Field theory and social science.* New York: Harper.

Lewis, B. (1982). Tips on school security. *School Administrator, 30,* 12.

Lewis, W. W. (1982). Ecological factors in successful residential treatment. *Behavioral Disorders, 7,* 149–156.

Liebert, R. M., Neale, J. M., & Davidson, E. S. (1973). *The early window: Effects of television on children and youth.* Elmsford, NY: Pergamon Press.

Lightfoot, S. L. (1976). *A school in transition: Stories of struggles and hope.* Unpublished manuscript.

Lightfoot, S. L. (1978). *Worlds apart: Relationships between families and schools.* New York: Basic Books.

Lindblad-Goldberg, M., & Dukes, J. (1985). Social support in black, low-income single-parent families: Normative and dysfunctional patterns. *American Journal of Orthopsychiatry, 55,* 42–58.

Linney, J. A., & Seidman, E. (1989). The future of schooling. *American Psychologist, 44,* 336–340.

Loeber, R. (1982). The stability of antisocial and delinquent child behavior: A review. *Child Development, 53,* 1431–1446.

Loeber, R., & Dishion, T. (1983). Early predictors of male delinquency: A review. *Psychological Bulletin, 94,* 68–99.

Lombard, T. (1979). Family-oriented emphasis for school psychologist: A needed orientation for training and professional practice. *Professional Psychology, 10,* 687–696.

Long, N. (1966). *Direct help to the classroom teacher.* Washington, DC: Washington School of Psychiatry.

Lorion, R. P. (1983). Evaluating preventive interventions: Guidelines for the serous social change agent. In R. D. Felner, L. Jason, J. Moritsugu, & S. S. Farber (Eds.), *Preventive psychology: Theory, research, and practice in community intervention* (pp. 251–268). New York: Pergamon Press.

Losen, S. N., & Diament, B. (1978). *Parent conferences in the schools. Procedures for developing effective partnership.* Boston: Allyn & Bacon.

Lovaas, O. I., Koegel, R., Simmons, J. Q., & Long, J. S. (1973). Some generalization and follow-up measures on autistic children in behavior therapy. *Journal of Applied Behavior Analysis, 6,* 131–166.

Lovaas, O. I., Schaeffer, B., & Simmons, J. (1965). Building social behavior in autistic children by use of electric shock. *Journal of Experimental Research in Personality, 1,* 99–109.

Loven, M. (1978). Four alternative approaches to the family/school liaison role. *Psychology in the Schools, 15,* 553–559.

Lowen, A. (1967). *The betrayal of the body.* New York: Macmillan.

Lowen, A., & Lowen, L. (1977). *The way to vibrant health: A manual of bioenergetic exercises.* New York: Harper & Row.

Lundquist, G. W. (1982). Needs assessment in organizational development. In C. R. Reynolds & T. B. Gutkin (Eds.), *The handbook of school psychology* (pp. 936–968). New York: Wiley.

Lutzker, J. R., Wesch, D., & Rice, J. M. (1984). A review of "Project 12-Ways": An ecobehavioral approach to the treatment and prevention of child abuse and neglect. *Advances in Behavior Research and Therapy, 6,* 63–73.

Mace, F. C., Page, T. J., Ivancic, M. T., & O'Brien, S. (1986). Effectiveness of brief time-out with and without contingent delay. *Journal of Applied Behavior Analysis, 19,* 79–86.

Madsen, C. J., Becker, W. C., & Thomas, D. R. (1968). Rules, praise, and ignoring: Elements of elementary classroom control. *Journal of Applied Behavior Analysis, 1,* 139–150.

Mahoney, M. J. (1974). *Cognition and behavior modification.* Cambridge, MA: Ballinger.

Mahoney, M. J. (1977). Reflections on the cognitive learning trend in psychotherapy. *American Psychologist, 32,* 5–13.

Mahoney, M. J., & Nezworski, S. (1985). Cognitive–behavioral approaches to children's problems. *Journal of Abnormal Child Psychology, 13,* 467–476.

Maller, J. B. (1929). *Cooperation and competition: An experimental study in motivation.* New York: Teachers College, Columbia University.

Manaster, G. J. (1977). *Adolescent development and the life tasks.* Boston: Allyn & Bacon.

Mancuso, W. A. (1983). Take these steps to keep schools safe and secure. *Executive Educator, 5,* 24–25, 27.

Mandler, G. (1954). Transfer of training as a function of degree of response overlearning. *Journal of Experimental Psychology, 47,* 411–417.

Mansfield, W., Alexander, D., & Farris, E. (1991). *Teacher survey on safe, disciplined and drug free schools.* Washington, DC: National Center for Education Statistics.

Martin, J. M. (1961). *Juvenile vandalism: A study of its nature and prevention.* Springfield, IL: C. C. Thomas.

Marvin, M., McCann, R., Connolly, J., Temkin, S., & Henning, P. (1977). Current activities in schools. In J. M. McPartland & E. L. McDill (Eds.), *Violence in schools.* Lexington, MA: Lexington Books.

Maslow, A. H. (1968). *Toward a psychology of being.* New York: Van Nostrand.

Mattick, H. W., & Caplan, N. S. (1962). *Chicago Youth Development Project: The Chicago Boys Club.* Ann Arbor, MI: Institute for Social Research.

Maultsby, M. C., Knipping, P., & Carpenter, L. (1974). Teaching self-help in the classroom with rational self-counseling. *Journal of School Health, 44,* 445–448.

Maultsby, M. C. (1971). *Handbook of rational self counseling.* Lexington, KY: University of Kentucky.

Maultsby, M. C. (1975). Rational behavior therapy for acting-out adolescents. *Social Casework, 56,* 35–43.

Maurer, A. (1974). Corporal punishment. *American Psychologist, 29,* 614–626.

Maxson, C. L., & Klein, M. W. (1983). Gangs, why we couldn't stay away. In J. R. Kleugel (Ed.), *Evaluating juvenile justice.* Newbury Park, CA: Sage.

Mayer, G. R., & Sulzer-Azaroff, B. (1991). Interventions for vandalism. In G. Stoner, M. R. Shinn, & H. M. Walker (Eds.), *Interventions for achievement and behavior problems.* Silver Springs, MD: National Association of School Psychologists.

McCord, W., & McCord, J. (1959). *Origins of crime: A new evaluation of the Cambridge–Somerville study.* New York: Columbia University Press.

McCord, W., McCord, J., & Howard, A. (1963). Familial correlates of aggression in nondelinquent male children. *Journal of Abnormal and Social Psychology, 62,* 79–93.

McCorkle, L., Elias, A., & Bixby, F. (1958). *The Highfields story: A unique experiment in the treatment of juvenile delinquency.* New York: Holt.

McCormack, S. (1981). To make discipline work, turn kids into self-managers. *Executive Educator, 3,* 26–27.

McDermott, M. J. (1979). *Criminal victimization in urban schools.* Albany, NY: Criminal Justice Research Center.

McGinnis, E., & Goldstein, A. P. (1984). *Skillstreaming the elementary school child: A guide for teaching prosocial skills.* Champaign, IL: Research Press.

McGinnis, E., & Goldstein, A. P. (1990). *Skillstreaming in early childhood.* Champaign, IL: Research Press.

McMullin, R., & Casey, B. (1974). *Talk sense to yourself.* Denver: Creative Social Designs.

McPartland, J. M., & McDill, E. L. (1977). *Violence in schools: Perspectives, programs, and positions.* Lexington, MA: Lexington Books, D. C. Heath.

Medway, F. J., & Smith, R. C., Jr. (1978). An examination of contemporary elementary school affective education programs. *Psychology in the Schools, 15*, 260–269.

Meichenbaum, D. H. (1977). *Cognitive–behavior modification: An integrative approach.* New York: Plenum Press.

Meichenbaum, D. H., & Asarnow, J. (1979). Cognitive–behavioral modification and metacognitive development: Implications for the classroom. In P. C. Kendall & S. D. Hollon (Eds.), *Cognitive–behavioral interventions: Theory, research, and procedures.* New York: Academic Press.

Meichenbaum, D. H., & Burland, S. (1979). Cognitive behavior modification with children. *School Psychology Digest, 8*, 426–433.

Meichenbaum, D. H., & Goodman, J. (1969). Reflection–impulsivity and verbal control of motor behavior. *Child Development, 40*, 785–797.

Meier, R. (1976). The new criminology: Continuity in criminological theory. *Journal of Criminal Law and Criminology, 67*, 461–469.

Meltzer, M. (1980). *The Chinese Americans.* New York: Thomas Y. Crowell.

Miller, D. (1986). Affective disorders and violence in adolescents. *Hospital and Community Psychiatry, 37*, 591–596.

Miller, G., & Prinz, R. J. (1991). Designing interventions for stealing. In G. Stoner, M. R. Shinn, & H. M. Walker (Eds.), *Interventions for achievement and behavior problems.* Silver Springs, MD: National Association of School Psychologists.

Miller, W. B. (1958). Lower class culture as a generation milieu of gang delinquency. *Journal of Social Issues, 14*, 5–19.

Miller, W. B. (1974). American youth gangs: Past and present. In A. Blumberg (Ed.), *Current perspectives on criminal behavior.* New York: Knopf.

Miller, W. B. (1975). *Violence by youth gangs and youth groups as a crime problem in major American cities.* Washington, DC: National Institute for Juvenile Justice and Delinquency Prevention.

Miller, W. B. (1980). Gangs, groups, and serious youth crime. In D. Shicker & D. H. Kelly (Eds.), *Critical issues in juvenile delinquency.* Lexington, MA: Lexington Books.

Miller, W. B. (1982). *Crime by youth gangs and groups in the United States.* Washington, DC: National Institute of Juvenile Justice and Delinquency Prevention.

Miller, W. B. (1990). Why the United States has failed to solve its youth gang problem. In C. R. Huff (Ed.), *Gangs in America.* Newbury Park, CA: Sage.

Mirande, A. (1987). *Gringo justice.* Notre Dame, IN: University of Notre Dame.

Miltenberger, R., & Fuqua, R. (1981). Overcorrection: A review and critical analysis. *Behavior Analyst, 4*, 123–141.

Moles, O. C. (1991, Winter). Student misconduct and intervention. *School Safety*, pp. 4–7.

Moleski, R., & Tosi, S. (1976). Comparative psychotherapy: Rational–emotive therapy versus systematic desensitization in the treatment of stuttering. *Journal of Consulting and Clinical Psychology, 44,* 309–311.

Moore, J. W., Garcia, R., Garcia, C., Cerda, L., & Valencia, F. (1978). *Homeboys, gangs, drugs, and prison in the barrios of Los Angeles.* Philadelphia: Temple University Press.

Moore, J. W., Vigil, D., & Garcia, R. (19983). Residence and territoriality in Chicano gangs. *Social Problems, 31,* 182–194.

Morales, A. (1981). *Treatment of Hispanic gang members.* Los Angeles: Neuropsychiatric Institute, University of California.

Moriarty, A. E., & Toussieng, P. W. (1976). *Adolescent coping.* New York: Grune & Stratton.

Morine-Dershimer, G. (1978-1979). Planning in classroom reality, an in-depth look. *Educational Research Quarterly, 3,* 83–99.

Morris, R. J. (1976). *Behavior modification with children.* Cambridge, MA: Winthrop.

Morrison, R. L., & Bellack, A. S. (1981). The role of social perception in social skills. *Behavior Therapy, 12,* 69–79.

Morse, W. C. (1974). Personal perspective. In J. M. Kauffman & C. D. Lewis (Eds.), *Teaching children with behavior disorders.* Columbus, OH: Merrill.

Morse, W. C., Smith, J. M., & Acker, N. (1977). *The psychodynamic approach: A self-instructional module* (Mimeo and videotape training packages). Ann Arbor: School of Education, University of Michigan.

Mowrer, O. H., & Mowrer, W. A. (1938). Enuresis: A method for its study and treatment. *American Journal of Orthopsychiatry, 8,* 436–447.

Mulvihill, D. J., Tumin, M. M., & Curtis, L. A. (1969). *Crimes of violence.* Washington, DC: National Commission on the Causes and Prevention of Violence.

Naranjo, C., & Ornstein, R. E. (1971). *On the psychology of meditation.* New York: Viking Press.

National Association of School Security Directors. (1975). *Crime in schools: 1974.* Washington, DC: Author.

National Center for Education Statistics. (1992). *Public school principal survey on safe, disciplined, and drug-free schools.* Washington, DC: U.S. Department of Education.

National Coalition on Television Violence. (1990, July–September). *NCTV News,* 2.

National Committee for Citizens in Education (1975). *Violence in our schools: What to know about it — What to do about it.* Columbia, MD: Author.

National Education Association. (1956). Teacher opinion on pupil behavior, 1955–1956. *Research Bulletin on the National Education Association, 34*(2).

National School Resource Network. (1980). *School violence prevention manual.* Cambridge, MA: Oelgeschlayer, Gunn & Hain.

Needle, J. A. & Stapleton, W. V. (1982). *Police handling of youth gangs.* Washington, DC: National Juvenile Justice Assessment Center.

Neill, S. B. (1978). Violence and vandalism: Dimensions and correctives. *Phi Delta Kappan, 59,* 302–307.

Nelson, C., & Rutherford, R. (1983). Time-out revisisted: Guidelines for its use in special education. *Exceptional Education Quarterly, 3,* 56–67.

Nemeroff, C. J., & Karoly, P. (1991). Operant methods. In F. H. Kanfer & A. P. Goldstein (Eds.), *Helping people change.* New York: Pergamon Press.

New Jersey Commissioner's Report to the Education Committee. (1988). Trenton.

New York State Task Force on Juvenile Gangs. (1990). *Reaffirming prevention.* Albany: Division for Youth.

Newcomer, P. L. (1980). *Understanding and teaching emotionally disturbed children.* Boston: Allyn & Bacon.

Newsom, C., Favell, J. E., & Rincover, A. (1982). *The effects and side effects of punishment on human behavior.* New York: Academic Press.

Novaco, R. W. (1975). *Anger control: The development and evaluation of an experimental treatment.* Lexington, MA: Lexington Books.

Nowakowski, R. (1966). *Vandals and vandalism in the schools: An analysis of vandalism in large school systems and a description of 93 vandals in Dade County schools.* Unpublished doctoral dissertation, University of Miami.

O'Leary, K. D., & Becker, W. C. (1967). Behavior modification of an adjustment class: A token reinforcement program. *Exceptional Children, 33,* 637–642.

O'Leary, K. D., Becker, W. C., Evans, M. B., & Saudargas, R. A. (1969). A token reinforcement program in a public school: A replication and systematic analyses. *Journal of Applied Behavior Analysis, 2,* 3–13.

O'Leary, K. D., Kaufman, K. F., Kass, R. E., & Drabman, R. S. (1970). The effects of loud and soft reprimands on the behavior of disruptive students. *Exceptional Children, 37,* 145–155.

O'Leary, K. D., & O'Leary, S. G. (1980). *Classroom management.* New York: Pergamon Press.

O'Leary, K. D., & Wilson, G. T. (1975). *Behavior therapy: Application and outcome.* Englewood Cliffs, NJ: Prentice-Hall.

O'Leary, S. G., & O'Leary, K. D. (1976). Behavior modification in the school. In H. Leitenberg (Ed.), *Handbook of behavior modification and behavior therapy.* Englewood Cliffs, NJ: Prentice-Hall.

Olds, D. L. (1984). *Final report: Prenatal/early infancy project.* Washington, DC: Maternal and Child Health Research, National Institute of Health.

Olsen, K. H., & Work, W. C. (1986, August). *Refinements in the curriculum and evaluation of a social problem solving program.* Paper presented at the annual meeting of the American Psychological Association, Washington, DC.

Orlick, T. (1978a). *Winning through cooperation.* Washington, DC: Acropolis.

Orlick, T. (1978b). *The cooperative sports and games book.* New York: Pantheon.

Orlick, T. (1982). *The second cooperative sports and games book.* New York: Pantheon.

Osborn, S. G., & West, D. J. (1979). Conviction records of fathers and sons compared. *British Journal of Criminology, 19,* 120–133.

Osgood, C. E. (1953). *Method and theory in experimental psychology.* New York: Oxford University Press.

Ossorio, P. (1973). Never smile at a crocodile. *Journal of Theory of Social Behavior, 3,* 121–140.

Partington, J. A., & Hinchcliffe, G. (1979). Some aspects of classroom management. *British Journal of Teacher Education, 5,* 231–241.

Patterson, G. R. (1965). A learning theory approach to the treatment of the school phobic child. In L. P. Ullmann & L. Krasner (Eds.), *Case studies in behavior modification.* New York: Holt, Rinehart, & Winston.

Patterson, G. R. (1982). *A social learning approach: 3. coercive family process.* Eugene, OR: Castalia.

Patterson, G. R. (1986). Performance models for antisocial boys. *American Psychologist, 41,* 432–444.

Patterson, G. R., & Anderson, D. (1964). Peers as social reinforcers. *Child Development, 35,* 951–960.

Patterson, G. R., Cobb, J. A., & Ray, R. S. (1973). A social engineering technology for retraining the families of aggressive boys. In H. E. Adams & I. P. Unikel (Eds.), *Issues and trends in behavior therapy.* Springfield, IL: C. C. Thomas.

Patterson, G. R., DeBaryshe, B. D., & Ramsey, E. (1989). A developmental perspective on antisocial behavior. *American Psychologist, 44,* 329–335.

Patterson, G. R., & Dishion, T. J. (1988). Multilevel family process models: Traits, interactions, and relationships. In R. Hinde & J. Stevenson-Hinde (Eds.), *Relationships within families: Mutual influences* (pp. 283–310). Oxford: Clarendon Press.

Patterson, G. R., Ray, R., & Shaw, D. (1968). *Direct intervention in families of deviant children.* Unpublished manuscript, University of Oregon.

Patterson, G. R., & Reid, J. B. (1973). Reciprocity and coercion: Two facets of social systems. In C. Neurenger & J. Meichael (Eds.), *Behavior modification in clinical psychology.* New York: Appleton-Century-Crofts.

Patterson, G. R., Reid, J. B., & Dishion, T. J. (1990). *Antisocial boys.* Eugene, OR: Castalia.

Patterson, G. R., Reid, J. B., Jones, R. R., & Conger, R. E. (1975). *A social learning approach to family intervention* (Vol. 1). Eugene, OR: Castalia.

Pazulinec, R., Meyerrose, M., & Sajwaj, T. (1983). Punishment via response cost. In S. Axelrod & J. Apsche (Eds.), *The effects of punishment on human behavior.* New York: Academic Press.

Pedersen, P. (1988). *A handbook for developing multicultural awareness.* Alexandria, VA: American Association for Counseling and Development.

Pelligrini, D. S., & Urbain, E. S. (1985). An evaluation of interpersonal cognitive problem solving training with children. *Journal of Child Psychology and Psychiatry, 26,* 17–41.

Pepitone, E. A. (1985). Children in cooperation and competition: Antecedents and consequences of self-orientation. In R. Slavin (Ed.), *Learning to cooperate, cooperating to learn.* New York: Plenum Press.

Pereira, G. J. (1978). *Teaching empathy through skill building versus interpersonal anxiety reduction methods.* Unpublished doctoral dissertation. Catholic University of America, Washington, DC.

Perlmutter, R. A. (1986). Emergency psychiatry and the family: The decision to admit. *Journal of Marital and Family Therapy, 12,* 153–162.

Perry, M. A., & Furukawa, M. J. (1980). Modeling methods. In F. H. Kanfer & A. P. Goldstein (Eds.), *Helping people change* (2nd ed.). New York: Pergamon Press.

Pesso, A. (1969). *Movement in psychotherapy.* New York: New York University Press.

Peterson, P. L., & Clark, C. M. (1978). Teacher's reports of their cognitive processes during teaching. *American Educational Research Journal, 15,* 555–565.

Pfiffner, L. J., Rosen, L. A., & O'Leary, S. G. (1985). The efficacy of an all-positive approach to classroom management. *Journal of Applied Behavior Analysis, 18,* 257–261.

Pilisuk, M. (1982). Delivery of social support: The social inoculation. *American Journal of Orthopsychiatry, 52,* 20–31.

Pines, M. (1979, January). Superkids. *Psychology Today,* pp. 53–63.

Pinkston, E. M., Reese, N. M., LeBlanc, J. M., & Baer, D. M. (1973). Independent control of a preschool child's aggression and peer interaction by contingent teacher attention. *Journal of Applied Behavior Analysis, 6,* 115–124.

Plath, K. (1965). *Schools within schools: A study of high school organization.* New York: Teachers College, Columbia University.

Plomin, R., Pedersen, N. L., McClearn, G. E., Nesselroade, J. R., & Bergeman, C. S. (1988). EAS temperaments during the last half of the life span: Twins reared apart and twins reared together. *Psychology and Aging, 3,* 43–50.

Plomin, R. (1989). Environment and genes: Determinants of behavior. *American Psychologist, 44,* 105–111.

Polk, K., & Schaeffer, W. E. (1972). *Schools and delinquency.* Englewood Cliffs, NJ: Prentice-Hall.

President's Commission on Law Enforcement and Administration of Justice. (1967). *Juvenile delinquency and youth crime.* Washington, DC: U.S. Government Printing Office.

Puffer, J. A. (1912). *The boy and his gangs.* Boston: Houghton Mifflin.

Purkey, S. C., & Smith, M. S. (1983). Effective schools: A review. *Elementary School Journal, 83,* 427–452.

Putka, G. (1991, April 12). Combatting gangs: As fears are driven from the classroom, students start to learn. *The Wall Street Journal,* pp. 1, 8.

Quicker, J. S. (1983). *Seven decades of gangs.* Sacramento: State of California Commission on Crime Control and Violence Prevention.

Ramirez, M. (1983). *Psychology of the Americas.* New York: Pergamon Press.

Rapport, M., Murphy, A., & Bailey, J. (1982). Ritalin vs response cost in the control of hyperactive children. *Journal of Applied Behavior Analysis, 15,* 205–216.

Rascon, A., Jr. (1981). Using security agents to enforce the law in your schools. *Thrust for Educational Leadership, 11,* 15–17.

Reckless, W. C. (1961). *The crime problem.* New York: Appleton-Century-Crofts.

Redl, F. (1959). The concept of the life-space interview. *American Journal of Orthopsychiatry, 29,* 1–18.

Redl, F. (1969, September). Aggression in the classroom. *Today's Education,* 30–32.

Redl, F., & Wineman, D. (1957). *The aggressive child.* Glencoe, IL: Free Press.

Reich, W. (1949). *Character analysis.* New York: Farrar, Straus & Giroux. (Original work published 1933)

Reid, J. B., & Patterson, G. R. (1991). Early prevention and intervention with conduct problems: A social interactional model for the integration of research and practice. In G. Stoner, M. R. Shinn, & H. M. Walker (Eds.), *Interventions for achievement and behavior problems.* Silver Springs, MD: National Association of School Psychologists.

Reid, W. H. (1985). The antisocial personality: A review. *Hospital and Community Psychiatry, 36,* 831–837.

Reinert, H. R. (1976). *Children in conflict: Educational strategies for the emotionally disturbed and behavior disordered.* St. Louis: C. V. Mosby.

Reuterman, N. A. (1975). Formal theories of gangs. In D. Cartwright, B. Tomson, & H. Schwartz (Eds.), *Gang delinquency.* Pacific Grove, CA: Brooks/Cole.

Rhodes, W. C. (1967). The disturbing child: A problem of ecological management. *Exceptional Children, 33,* 449–455.

Rhodes, W. C., & Gibbins, S. (1972). Community programming for the behaviorally deviant child. In H. Quay & J. Werry (Eds.), *Psychopathological disorders of childhood.* New York: Wiley.

Richards, P. (1976). *Patterns of middle class vandalism: A case study of suburban adolescence.* Doctoral dissertation, Northwestern University.

Rickel, A. U., Eshelman, A. K., & Loigman, G. A. (1983). Social problem solving training: A follow-up study of cognitive and behavioral effects. *American Journal of Community Psychology, 11,* 15–28.

Risley, T. R. (1977). The social context of self-control. In R. Stuart (Ed.), *Behavioral self-management.* New York: Brunner/Mazel.

Robins, L. N., & Earls, F. (1985). A program for preventing antisocial behavior for high-risk infants and preschoolers: A research prospectus. In R. L. Hough, P. A. Gongla, V. B. Brown, & S. E. Goldston (Eds.), *Psychiatric epidemiology and prevention: The possibilities* (pp. 73–84). Los Angeles: Neuropsychiatric Institute.

Robins, L. N., & Ratcliff, L. S. (1979). Risk factors in the continuation of childhood antisocial behavior into adulthood. *International Journal of Mental Health, 7*(3–4), 96–116.

Robins, L. N., West, P. A., & Herjanic, B. L. (1975). Arrests and delinquency in two generations: A study of black urban families and their children. *Journal of Child Psychology and Psychiatry, 16,* 125–140.

Rogers, C. R. (1957). The necessary and sufficient conditions of therapeutic personality change. *Journal of Consulting Psychology, 21,* 95–103.

Rolf, I. (1977). *Rolfing: The integration of human structures.* Boulder, CO: The Rolf Institute.

Rosenberg, M. (1975). The dissonant context and the adolescent self-concept. In S. E. Dragastin & G. H. Elder (Eds.), *Adolescence in the life cycle.* Washington, DC: Hemisphere.

Rosenberg, M. S., & Reppucci, N. D. (1985). Primary prevention of child abuse. *Journal of Consulting and Clinical Psychology, 53,* 576–585.

Rothenberg, B. B. (1970). Children's social sensitivity and the relationship to interpersonal competence, interpersonal comfort, and intellectual level. *Developmental Psychology, 2,* 335–350.

Roush, D. W. (1984, January). Rational-emotive therapy and youth: Some new techniques for counselors. *Personnel and Guidance Journal,* pp. 223–227.

Rubel, R. J. (1977). *Unruly school: Disorders, disruptions, and crimes.* Lexington, MA: D. C. Heath.

Rutherford, W. L. (1985). School principals as effective leaders. *Phi Delta Kappan, 67,* 31–34.

Rutter, M. (1983). School effects on pupil progress: Research findings and policy implications. *Child Development, 54,* 1–29.

Rutter, M., & Giller, H. (1983). *Juvenile delinquency: Trends and perspectives.* New York: Penguin Books.

Rutter, M., Maughan, B., Mortimore, P., & Ouston, J. (1979). *Fifteen thousand hours: Secondary schools and their effects on children.* Cambridge, MA: Harvard University Press.

Sabers, D. S., Cushing, K. S., & Berliner, D. C. (1991). Differences among teachers in a task characterized by simultaneity, multidimensimality, and immediacy. *American Educational Research Journal, 28,* 63–88.

Safer, D. J., & Allen, R. P. (1976). *Hyperactive children. Diagnosis and management.* Baltimore: University Park Press.

Sajwaj, T., Culver, P., Hall, C., & Lehr, L. (1972). Three simple punishment techniques for the control of classroom disruptions. In G. Semb (Ed.), *Behavior analysis and education.* Lawrence, KS: University of Kansas.

Sallend, S., & Allen, E. (1985). Comparative effects of externally managed and self-managed response cost system on inappropriate classroom behavior. *Journal of School Psychology, 23,* 59–67.

Sallis, J. (1983). Aggressive behavior of children: A review of behavioral intervention and future directions. *Education and Treatment of Children, 6,* 175–191.

Sandler, J., & Steele, H. V. (1991). Aversion methods. In F. H. Kanfer & A. P. Goldstein (Eds.), *Helping people change.* New York: Pergamon Press.

Sarason, I. G. (1968). Verbal learning, modeling, and juvenile delinquency. *American Psychologist, 23,* 254–266.

Sarason, I. G., Glaser, E. M., & Fargo, G. A. *Reinforcing productive classroom behavior.* New York: Behavioral.

Sarason, I. G., & Sarason, B. R. (1981). Teaching cognitive and social skills to high school students. *Journal of Consulting and Clinical Psychology, 49,* 908–918.

Sarason, S. B. (1982). *The culture of the school and the problem of change* (2nd ed.). Boston: Allyn & Bacon.

Sarason, S. B., Zitnay, G., & Grossman, F. K. (1971). *The creation of a community setting.* Syracuse, NY: Syracuse University.

School Safety Council. (1989). *Weapons in schools.* Washington, DC: Department of Justice.

Schwartz, B. N., & Disch, R. (1970). *White racism.* New York: Dell.

Schwitzgebel, R. (1964). *Street corner research: An experimental approach to the juvenile delinquent.* Cambridge, MA: Harvard University Press.

Seidman, E. (1988). Back to the future, community psychology: Unfolding a theory of social intervention. *American Journal of Community Psychology, 16,* 3–24.

Selman, R. L. (1980). *The growth of interpersonal understanding: Developmental and clinical analyses.* New York: Academic Press.

Sennett, R. (1980). *Authority.* New York: Knopf.

Sewell, E., McCoy, J. F., & Sewell, W. R. (1973). Modification of antagonistic social behavior using positive reinforcement for other behavior. *Psychological Record, 23,* 499–504.

Sexton, P. C. (1967). *The American school: A sociological perspective.* Englewood Cliffs, NJ: Prentice-Hall.

Sharan, S., Raviv, S., & Russell, P. L. (1982). *Cooperative and traditional classroom learning and the cooperative behavior of seventh-grade pupils in mixed-ethnic classrooms.* Unpublished manuscript, University of Tel-Aviv, Israel.

Sharp, K. C. (1981). Impact of interpersonal problem-solving training on preschoolers' social competency. *Journal of Applied Developmental Psychology*, 2, 129-143.

Shavelson, R. J. (1973). What is the basic teaching skill? *Journal of Teacher Education*, 24, 144-147.

Shavelson, R. J. (1976). Teachers' decision making. In N. L. Gage (Ed.), *The psychology of teaching methods: The seventy-fifth yearbook of the National Society for the Study of Education, Part I.* Chicago: University of Chicago Press.

Shavelson, R. J., & Stern, P. (1981). Research on teachers' pedagogical thoughts, judgments, decisions, and behavior. *Review of Educational Research, 51*, 455-498.

Shaw, C. R., & McKay, H. D. (1942). *Juvenile delinquency and urban areas: A study of rates of delinquents in relation to differential characteristics of local communities in American cities.* Chicago: University of Chicago Press.

Sherman, J. A. (1965). Use of reinforcement and imitation to reinstate verbal behavior in mute psychotics. *Journal of Abnormal Psychology, 70*, 155-164.

Shore, E., & Sechrest, L. (1961). Concept attainment as a function of number of positive instances presented. *Journal of Educational Psychology, 52*, 303-307.

Short, J. F. (1990). New wine in old bottles? Change and continuity in American gangs. In C. R. Huff (Ed.), *Gangs in America.* Newbury Park, CA: Sage.

Shulman, L. A., & Elstein, A. S. (1975). Studies of problem solving, judgment, and decision making: Implications for educational research. In F. N. Kerlinger (Ed.), *Review of research in education* (Vol. 3). Itasca, IL: Peacock.

Shure, M. B., & Spivack, G. (1979). Interpersonal problem solving, thinking, and adjustment in the mother-child dyad. In M. W. Kent & J. E. Rolf (Eds.), *Social competence in children* (pp. 201-219). Hanover, NH: University Press of New England.

Siegel, L. M., & Senna, J. J. (1991). *Juvenile delinquency: Theory, practice and law.* St. Paul: West.

Silberman, C. E. (1970). *Crisis in the classroom.* New York: Vintage Books.

Silverstein, B., & Krate, R. (1975). *Children of the dark ghetto.* New York: Praeger.

Simmons, R. G., Burgeson, R., Carlton-Ford, S., & Blyth, D. A. (1987). The impact of cumulative change in early adolescence. *Child Development, 58*, 1220-1234.

Singh, N. N. (1987). Overcorrection of oral reading errors. *Behavior Modification, 11*, 165-181.

Sizer, T. (1984). *Horace's compromise: The dilemma of the American high school.* Boston: Houghton-Mifflin.

Skinner, B. F. (1938). *The behavior of organisms: An experimental analysis.* New York: Appleton-Century-Crofts.

Skinner, B. F. (1953). *Science and human behavior.* New York: Macmillan.

Skogan, W. G. (1989). Social change and the future of violent crime. In T. R. Gurr (Ed.), *Violence in America: Vol. 1. The history of crime.* Newbury Park, CA: Sage.

Slavin, R. E. (1980). *Using student team learning* (rev. ed). Baltimore, MD: Center for Social Organization of Schools, Johns Hopkins University.

Slavin, R. E., Leavey, M., & Madden, N. A. (1982, April). *Effects of student teams and individualized instruction on student mathematics achievement, attitudes, and behaviors.* Paper presented at the meeting of the American Educational Research Association, New York.

Slavin, R., Sharan, S., Kagan, S., Hertz-Lazarowitz, R., Webb, C. & Schmuck, R. (1985). *Learning to cooperate, cooperating to learn.* New York: Plenum Press.

Slavson, S. R. (1964). *A testbook in analytic group psychotherapy.* New York: International Universities Press.

Smith, C. (1982). Use these strategies for stronger school security. *Executive Educator, 4,* 21–22.

Smith, H. C. (1973). *Sensitivity training.* New York: McGraw-Hill.

Snyder, J. J. (1977). Reinforcement analysis of interaction in problem and non-problem families. *Journal of Abnormal Psychology, 86,* 528–535.

Snyder, J. J., & Patterson, G. R. (1986). The effects of consequences on patterns of social interaction: A quasi-experimental approach to reinforcement of natural interaction. *Child Development, 57,* 1257–1268.

Solomon, E. (1977). *Structured learning therapy with abusive parents: Training in self-control.* Unpublished doctoral dissertation, Syracuse University, Syracuse, NY.

Soriano, F. I., & De La Rosa, M. R. (1990). Cocaine use and criminal activities among Hispanic juvenile delinquents in Florida. In R. Glick & J. Moore (Eds.), *Drugs in Hispanic communities.* New Brunswick, NJ: Rutgers University Press.

Soriano, F. I. (1993). Cultural sensitivity and gang interventions. In A. P. Goldstein & C. H. Huff (Eds.), *The gang intervention handbook.* Champaign, IL: Research Press.

Spence, S. H. (1981). Differences in social skills performance between institutionalized juvenile male offenders and a comparable group of boys without offense records. *British Journal of Clinical Psychology, 20,* 163–171.

Spergel, I. (1965). *Street gang work: Theory and practice.* New York: Addison-Wesley.

Spergel, I. A., Ross, R. E., Curry, G. D., & Chance, R. (1989). *Youth gangs: Problem and response.* Washington, DC: Office of Juvenile Justice and Delinquency Prevention.

Spivack, G., Platt, J. J., & Shure, M. B. (1976). *The problem-solving approach to adjustment.* San Francisco: Jossey-Bass.

Spivack, G., & Shure, M. B. (1974). *Social adjustment in young children.* San Francisco: Jossey-Bass.

Stallings, J. (1975). Implementation and child effects of teaching practices in follow through classroom. *Monograph of the Society for Research in Child Development, 40*(7–8), Serial No. 163.

Stark, E., & Flitcraft, A. (1988). Violence among intimates. In V. B. Van Hasett (Ed.), *Handbook of family violence.* New York: Plenum Press.

Stephens, R. D. (1992, March). Gangs vs. schools: Assessing the score in your community. *School Safety Update,* p. 8.

Stephens, R. D. (1993). School-based interventions: Safety and security. In A. P. Goldstein & C. R. Huff (Eds.), *The gang intervention handbook.* Champaign, IL: Research Press.

Stephens, T. M. (1976). *Directive teaching of children with learning and behavioral handicaps.* Columbus, OH: Merrill.

Stinchcombe, A. L. (1964). *Rebellion in a high school.* Chicago: Quadrangle Books.

Straughan, J. (1968). The application of operant conditioning to the treatment of elective mutism. In H. N. Sloane, Jr. & B. A. MacAulay (Eds.), *Operant procedures in remedial speech and language training.* Boston: Houghton-Mifflin.

Strauss, M. A. (1977, 1978). Wife-beating: How common and why? *Victimology, 2,* 443–458.

Sturm, D. (1980). *Therapist aggression tolerance and dependence tolerance under standardized conditions of hostility an dependency.* Unpublished master's thesis, Syracuse University, Syracuse, NY.

Sue, D. W., & Sue, S. (1982). Cross-cultural counseling competencies. *The Counseling Psychologist, 19*(2), 45–52.

Sutherland, E. H. (1937). *Principles of criminology.* Philadelphia: J. B. Lippincott.

Sutherland, E. H., & Cressey, D. R. (1974). *Criminology.* New York: J. B. Lippincott.

Swap, S. M. (1974). Disturbing classroom behaviors: A developmental and ecological view. *Exceptional Children, 41,* 163–172.

Swap, S. M. (1978). The ecological model of emotional disturbance in children: A status report and proposed synthesis. *Behavioral Disorders, 3,* 186–196.

Swap, S. M. (1987). *Enhancing parent involvement in schools.* New York: Teachers College, Columbia University Press.

Swap, S. M. (1992). Parent involvement and success for all children: What we know. In S. Christenson & J. C. Conoley (Eds.), *Home–school collaboration: building a fundamental educational resource.* Washington, DC: National Association of School Psychologists.

Swap, S. M., Prieto, A. G., & Harth, R. (1982). Ecological perspectives of the emotionally disturbed child. In R. L. McDowell, G. W. Adamson, & F. H. Wood (Eds.), *Teaching emotionally disturbed children.* Boston: Little, Brown.

Sweeney, J. (1982). Research synthesis on effective school leadership. *Educational Leadership, 39,* 346–352.

Tannenbaum, R. (1939). *Crime and the community.* New York: Columbia University Press.

Tharp, R. G., & Wetzel, R. J. (1969). *Behavior modification in the natural environment.* New York: Academic Press.

Thomas, A., & Chess, S. (1977). *Temperament and development.* New York: Brunner/Mazel.

Thomas, A., Chess, S., & Birch, H. (1968). *Temperament and behavior disorders in children.* New York: New York University Press.

Thomas, D. R., Becker, W. C., & Armstrong, M. (1968). Production and elimination of disruptive classroom behavior by systematically varying teacher's behavior. *Journal of Applied Behavior Analysis, 1,* 35–45.

Thomas, J. D., Presland, I. E., Grant, M. D., & Glynn, T. L. (1978). Natural rates of teacher approval and disapproval in grade-7 classrooms. *Journal of Applied Behavior Analysis, 11,* 91–94.

Thompson, D. W., & Jason, L. A. (1988). Street gangs and preventive interventions. *Criminal Justice and Behavior, 15,* 323–333.

Thorndike, E. L., & Woodworth, R. S. (1901). The influence of improvement in one mental function upon the efficieincy of other functions. *Psychological Review, 8,* 247–261.

Thrasher, F. M. (1963). *The gang.* Chicago: University of Chicago Press. (Original work published 1927)

Tosi, D. (1974). *Youth: Toward personal growth — a rational-emotive approach.* Columbus, OH: Merrill.

Tosi, D. C., Meeks, S., & Turk, L. M. (1982). Factors contributing to teacher stress: Implications for research, prevention, and remediation. *Behavioral Counseling Quarterly, 2,* 2–25.

Tracy, P. E. (1979). *Subcultural delinquency: A comparison of the incidence and seriousness of gang and nongang member offensivity.* Philadelphia: University of Pennsylvania Center for Studies in Criminology and Ciminal Law.

Travers, R. M. W. (1962). A study of the relationship of psychological research to educational practice. In R. Glaser (Ed.), *Training, research and education.* Pittsburgh: University of Pittsburgh.

Truax, C. B., Wargo, D. G., & Silber, L. D. (1966). Effects of group psychotherapy with high accurate empathy and nonpossessive warmth upon female institutionalized delinquents. *Journal of Abnormal Psychology, 71,* 267–274.

Tuma, J. M. (1990). Current status of insight oriented treatment with children. *Journal of Clinical Child Psychology.*

Underwood, B. J., & Schultz, R. W. (1960). *Meaningfulness and verbal behavior.* New York: J. B. Lippincott.

Unger, C. (1974). Treatment of deviance by the social welfare system: History and structure. In W. C. Rhodes & S. Head (Eds.), *A study of child variance: Service delivery systems* (Vol. 3). Ann Arbor, MI: Institute for the Study of Mental Retardation and Related Disabilities.

Urbain, E. S. (1980). *Interpersonal problem-solving training and social perspective taking with impulsive children via modeling, role play, and self instruction.* Unpublished doctoral dissertation, University of Minnesota.

Van Houton, R. (1982). Punishment: From the animal laboratory to the applied setting. In S. Axelrod & J. Apsche (Eds.), *The effects and side effects of punishment on human behavior.* New York: Academic Press.

Van Houten, R., Daley, D. (1983). Are social reprimands effective? In S. Axelrod & J. Apsche (Eds.), *The effects of punishment on human behavior.* New York: Academic Press.

Van Houten, R., Nau, P., McKenzie-Keating, S., Sameoto, D., & Colavecchia, B. (1982). An analysis of some variables influencing the effectiveness of reprimands. *Journal of Applied Behavior Analysis, 15,* 65–83.

Vigil, J. D. (1983). Chicano gangs: One response to Mexican urban adaptation in the Los Angeles area. *Urban Anthropology, 12,* 45–75.

Vigil, J. D., & Long, J. M. (1990). Emic and etic perspectives on gang cultures: The Chicano case. In C. R. Huff (Ed.), *Gangs in America.* Newbury Park, CA: Sage.

Vorrath, H., & Brendtro, L. K. (1974). *Positive peer culture.* Chicago: Aldine.

Vukelich, R., & Hake, D. F. (1971). Reduction of dangerously aggressive behavior in a severely retarded resident through a combination of positive reinforcement procedures. *Journal of Applied Behavior Analysis, 4,* 215–225.

Wahler, R., & Fox, J. (1980). Solitary toy play and time out: A family treatment package for children with aggressive and oppositional behavior. *Journal of Applied Behavior Analysis, 14*, 327–338.

Wahler, R. G., & Pollio, H. R. (1968). Behavior and insight: A case study in behavior therapy. *Journal of Experimental Research in Personality, 3*, 45–56.

Wahler, R. G., Winkel, G. H., Peterson, R. F., & Morrison, D. C. (1965). Mothers as behavior therapists for their own children. *Behaviour Research and Therapy, 3*, 113–124.

Walker, C. E. (1975). *Learn to relax*. Englewood Cliffs, NJ: Spectrum Books.

Walker, H. M. (1979). *The acting-out child: Coping with classroom disruption*. Boston: Allyn & Bacon.

Walker, H. (1983). Applications of response cost in school settings: Outcomes, issues, and recommendations. *Exceptonal Education Quarterly, 3*, 47–55.

Walker, H. M., Hops, H., & Fiegenbaum, E. (1976). Deviant classroom behavior as a function of combinations of social and token reinforcement and cost contingency. *Behavior Therapy, 7*, 76–88.

Walker, H. M., Mattson, R. H., & Buckley, N. K. (1971). The function analysis of behavior within an experimental classroom setting. In W. C. Becker (Ed.), *An empirical basis for change in education*. Chicago: Science Research Associates.

Walker, H. M., Street, A., Garrett, B., & Crossen, J. (1977). *Experiments with response cost in playground and classroom settings*. Eugene, OR: Center at Oregon for Research in the Behavioral Education of the Handicapped, University of Oregon.

Wang, M. C., & Walberg, H. J. (1991). Teaching and educational effectiveness: Research synthesis and consensus from the field. In H. C. Waxman & H. N. Walberg (Eds.), *Effective teaching: Current research* (pp. 81–104). Berkeley, CA: McCutchan.

Ward, M. H., & Baker, B. L. (1968). Reinforcement therapy in the classroom. *Journal of Applied Behavior Analysis, 1*, 323–328.

Warren, R., Smith, G., & Velten, E. (1984). Rational–emotive therapy and the reduction of interpersonal anxiety in junior high school students. *Adolescents, 19*, 893–902.

Wasik, B., Senn, K., Welch, R. H., & Cooper, B. R. (1968). Behavior modification with culturally deprived school children: Two case studies. *Journal of Applied Behavior Analysis, 2*, 171–179.

Wattenberg, W. W., & Balistrieri, J. J. (1950). Gang membership and juvenile misconduct. *American Sociological Review, 15*, December.

Webster, R. E. (1976). A time-out procedure in a public school setting. *Psychology in the School, 13*, 72–76.

Webster's Encyclopedic Dictionary of the English Language. (1973). Chicago: Consolidated.

Weiner, B. (1979). A theory of motivation for some classroom experiences. *Journal of Educational Psychology, 71*, 3–25.

Weissberg, R. P., Gesten, E. L., Carnilce, C. L., Toro, P. A., Rapkin, B. D., Davidson, E., & Cowen, E. L. (1981a). Social problem-solving skills training: A competence building intervention with 2nd–4th grade children. *American Journal of Community Psychology, 9*, 411–424.

Weissberg, R. P., Gesten, E. L., Rapkin, B. D., Cowen, E. L., Davidson, E., Flores de Apondaca, R., & McKim, B. J. (1981b). The evaluation of a social problem-solving training program for suburban and inner city third grade children. *Journal of Consulting and Clinical Psychology, 49*, 251–261.

Welsh, R. S. (1978, July). Delinquency, corporal punishment and the schools. *Crime and Delinquency,* 336–354.

Wenk, E. A. (1975, August). Juvenile justice and the public schools; mutual benefit through educational reform. *Juvenile Justice,* pp. 7–14.

Werner, E. & Smith, R. (1982). *Vulnerable but invincible: A study of resilient children.* New York: McGraw-Hill.

Wesch, D., & Lutzker, J. R. (1991). A comprehensive 5-year evaluation of Project 12-Ways: An ecobehavioral program for treating and preventing child abuse and neglect. *Journal of Family Violence, 6,* 17–35.

West, J. F., & Idol, L. (1987). School consultation (Part 1): An interdisciplinary perspective on theory, models, and research. *Journal of Learning Disabilities, 20,* 388–408.

West, W. G. (1975). Adolescent deviance and the school. *Interchange, 6,* 49–55.

Wetzel, J. R. (1989, Winter). School crime: Annual statistical snapshot. *School Safety,* p. 8.

Wetzel, R. (1966). Use of behavior techniques in a case of compulsive stealing. *Journal of Consulting and Criminal Psychology, 30,* 367–374.

Whalen, C. K., Henker, B., & Hinshaw, S. P. (1985). Cognitive–behavioral therapies for hyperactive children: Premises, problems, and prospects. *Journal of Abnormal Child Psychology, 13,* 391–410.

White, J., & Fallis, A. (1981). *Vandalism prevention programs: A case study approach.* Toronto, Canada: Ontario Government Bookstore.

White, J. L. (1984). *The psychology of Blacks.* Englewood Cliffs, NJ: Prentice-Hall.

White, G. D., Nielson, G., & Johnson, S. M. (1972). Time out duration and the suppression of deviant behavior in children. *Journal of Applied Behavior Analysis, 5,* 111–120.

White, M. A. (1975). Natural rates of teacher approval and disapproval in the classroom. *Journal of Applied Behavior Analysis, 8,* 367–372.

Williams, D. R., Meyer, L. M., Harootunian, B. (1992). Introduction and implementation of cooperative learning in heterogeneous classrooms: Middle school teachers' perspectives. *Research in Middle Level Education, 16,* 115–130.

Wilson, J. Q., & Herrnstein, R. J. (1985). *Crime and human nature.* New York: Simon & Schuster.

Wilson, R. W. (1970). *Learning to be Chinese.* Cambridge, MA: MIT Press.

Winer, J. I., Hilpert, P. L., Gesten, E. L., Cowen, E. L., & Schubin, W. E. (1982). The evaluation of a kindergarten social problem solving program. *Journal of Primary Prevention, 2,* 205–216.

Witkin, G. (1991, April 8). Kids who kill. *U.S. News and World Report,* pp. 26–32.

Witt, J., & Elliott, S. (1982). The response cost lottery: A time efficient and effective classroom intervention. *Journal of School Psychology, 20,* 155–161.

Wolf, M., Risley, T., & Mees, H. (1964). Application of operant conditioning procedures to the behavior problems of an autistic child. *Behaviour Research and Therapy, 1,* 305–312.

Wynne, E. A. (1980). *Looking at schools: Good, bad, and indifferent.* Lexington, MA: Lexington Books.

Yablonsky, L. (1967). *The violent gang.* New York: Penguin Books.

Yankelovich, D. (1975). How students control their drug crisis. *Psychology Today, 9,* 39–42.

Young, H. (1975). Rational casework with adolescents. *Journal of School Social Work, 1,* 15–20.

Young, H. (1974). *A rational counseling primer.* New York: Institute for Rational Living.

Youth Violence. (1991, November 25). *New York Times,* p. 23.

Zelie, K., Stone, C. I., & Lehr, E. (1980). Cognitive–behavioral intervention in school discipline: A preliminary study. *Personnel and Guidance Journal, 59,* 80–83.

Zimmerman, D. (1983). Moral education. In A. P. Goldstein (Ed.), *Prevention and control of aggression.* New York: Pergamon Press.

Zimring, R. (1977). Determinants of the death rate from robbery. *Journal of Legal Studies, 6,* 317–332.

Zinsmeister, K. (1990, June). Growing up scared. *The Atlantic Monthly,* pp. 49–66.

Zwier, G., & Vaughn, G. M. (1984). Three ideological orientations in school vandalism research. *Review of Educational Research, 54,* 263–292.

Index

I

L

M

N

O

Observational methods, 80, 81
Open classrooms, 20
Oral development stage, 123
Out-of-home placement, 229–231
Overcorrection, 106
Overlearning, 48, 49
  in transfer facilitation, 111

P

Parent models, 71
Parent training
  in prevention programs, 25
  workshops, 225
Parents
  coercive communication, 226
  decision making, 225, 226
  school collaboration, 219–223
  volunteer programs, 224
Parents' Network of the National
  Committee for Citizen in
  Education, 221
Partial reinforcement, 87
Partnership programs, 232, 233
Passive aggression, 55
Peer influences, 72, 73
Peer models, 71
Performance feedback
  overview, 34, 35
  in skillstreaming groups, 47, 48
  use by trainers, 40
  videotaping in, 48
Personality factors
  psychodynamic theory, 122–125
  youth crime theory, 120, 121
Phallic developmental stage, 123
Physical environment factor, 206,
  207
Physical punishment (*see* Corporal
  punishment)
Physical restraint, 133, 134
Planned ignoring, 130 (*see also*
  Extinction)
Play therapy, 126
"Pleasure principle," 122, 135
Positive reinforcement
  in classroom contingency
    management, 82–85
  definition, 76

identification of, 82–85
prescriptive guidelines, 108, 109
presentation of, 86–90
preventive use of, 89
and time-out, 94
Praise, 88
Prepare Curriculum, 64–73
Prepared scripts, 57
Prescriptive strategies, 108, 109
  hierarchy of, 108, 109
  in preventive programs, 25, 26
  in schools, 204
Prevention, 17–26
  cognitive–behavioral approaches,
    21–26
  implementation, 18, 21
  multidimensional perspective, 204
  school-based programs, 19–26
  target levels, 18, 19
  teachers' efforts, 185
Primary prevention
  definition, 17
  implementation, 18
  school-based programs, 19–26,
    197
  target levels, 18, 19
Principals
  influence on discipline problems,
    202
  leadership style, 9, 202
  perception of discipline
    problems, 201, 202
Private schools, 10
"Problem frame," 191
Problem-solving groups, 225
Problem-solving training, 64, 65
Program planning, 129
Programmed generalization, 110,
  111
Progressive relaxation training,
  69
Prompting, 58
Property crimes (*see* Vandalism)
Psychodynamic interventions,
  120–145
  criticism of, 144, 145
  essential principles, 129
  surface behavior manipulations,
    129–135
  theoretical basis, 120–125
Psychoeducational approaches, 32,
  139, 140

explicit admission of problems
in, 201
versus families, violence cause,
199
and gangs, 156–166, 200
information transfer to families,
219–222
intervention programs, 19–26,
200–211
role in violence, 198–200
security measures, 200, 201
size of, 9
society's role, 200
system causes of violence, 198
tracking effects, 199
use as community centers, 225,
226
Secondary prevention, 17
"Security dads," 222
Security officers, 200
Self-actualization, 140
Self-reinforcement, 113
Shaping
in classroom contingency
management, 89, 90
prescriptive guidelines, 109
in skillstreaming groups, 57
Signal interference technique, 130
Silent alarm systems, 201
Situational perception training, 66,
68
Skillstreaming, 33–63
group organization in, 39–42
homework assignments, 50, 51
management problems, 53–62
origins, 33
preparation, 35–37
sessions in, 40–44
techniques, 33–35, 44–48
threat reduction methods, 58–60
trainee selection, 37
trainer selection and preparation,
35–37
and transfer of training, 48–51
SOAR program, 163
Social adjustment, 23
Social learning theory, 32
Social perception, 66, 68
Social problem solving
adjustment relationship, 23
and empathy level, 25
individualization of, 26

prescriptive use, 25
in school-based prevention
programs, 22–24
Social reinforcement
in classroom contingency
management, 82–84
identification of, 82, 84
pairing with praise, 88
performance feedback use, 47
Social skills (*see also* Skillstreaming)
in aggressive youth, 30, 31
Sociopathy, 155
Spontaneous recovery, 92, 93
Spouse abuse, 6
"Spring fever effects," 10
Stereotyping, 121
Strain theory, gang formation, 149
Street Club Project, 158
Stress management, 68, 69
Student victims, 8, 9
Subculture theory, gangs, 149
Suburban schools, 23
Superego concept, 122, 123
"Synomorphy," 215
Systematic Management Plan for
School Discipline, 197
Systems approach, 196, 216 (*see
also* Ecological perspective)

T

Tailored intervention (*see
Prescriptive strategies)
Teacher assault, 8, 9, 172
Teacher praise, 88, 109
Teacher–principal interactions, 12
Teacher–teacher interactions, 12
Teachers, 171–195
actions of, 190–193
adaptations of, 193
assessments of antisocial
behaviors, 194
collaboration with parents, 222,
223
communication with parents,
220
cue sensitivity, 186
decision making, 174–180, 195
developmental stages, 195
implicit theory of, 180–182
intentions of, 184, 185